CHOOSE: MISERY AND
ILLNESS OR
HEALTH AND HAPPINESS

PREVENTING BETTER THAN HEALING

Man is as good as his information
History of the Doctor

BY COBUS VAN DER MERWE

Other books by this author

82 SINS OF THE CHURCH
TO DO OR NOT TO DO
THE LOST TRIBES OF ISRAEL AND THE JEWS
EVERYTHING AND WHAT NOT
MERVIC TO MERWE 1600 YEARS
MY SHEEP HEAR MY VOICE
MY ROMANCES FROM LIZZIE TO MERCEDES

Index

Please note that the Bible is often referred to as —The Maker's Handbook.‖

INTRODUCTION

WASH YOUR HANDS —UNDER THE TAP‖

As children, when our game was going just fine only to be interrupted by mother's call, —Come on children, the food is on the table, wash your hands under the tap and come eat,‖ we always wondered whether the —hand washing‖ was really necessary since our hands seemed pretty clean to us. As the saying goes, —Mother knows best.‖

Now here in 3rd Millennium A.D. we are bombarded over the —ether‖ with warnings to wash our hands because of all sorts of epidemics, amongst others the H1N1 swine-flu virus. These warnings are not to be taken lightly, and when you see antiseptic dispensers against the walls of public places, and at your disposal, say thanks and utilize it for your protection. By reading this book you will come to know quite a few very important facts that relate to the prevention of diseases not only by keeping clean on the outside, but being —clean‖ in our eating habits, as well.

To my mind, one of our big problems is that people are people and people listen to people who talk about too many things they know too little about. And that is particularly true in politics, where quite often those that say the most know the least and visa versa. I will recommend a critical mind to all; it works every time it's tried. Proverbs 14:15 The simple believeth every word: but the prudent man looketh well to his going.

Hand washing is not a new concept, but has been a recorded practice for as far back as the time when the Twelve Tribes of Israel were trekking through, first, the Desert of Shur, then the Desert of Paran, then through the Desert of Sinai where the wonderful TEN COMMANDMENTS of the Almighty, written with His finger on slate tablets, were given to that all time great leader, Mozes. Finally they made the last trek through the Desert of Zin. We must bear in mind that General Mozes had to do with a population of circa 2 million.

In the old days, even in the time of the Messiah's visit on earth, it was essential to wash the hands before a meal. Water

5

was poured on the hands to create running water. I remember when I was a boy circa 80 years ago on the farm, how we washed our hands with water being poured on them before milking the cows.

The reader will undoubtedly find this book not only a very interesting read, but most informing that can help you live a healthy long life. The author, at the time of writing enjoys good health and has in over 83 years never had surgery or serious illnesses and still enjoys the use of all teeth, tonsils and appendix. Now if you should ask me what the secret is, I will say, —Its in the BOOK.‖

—Anything I can do, you can do better.‖

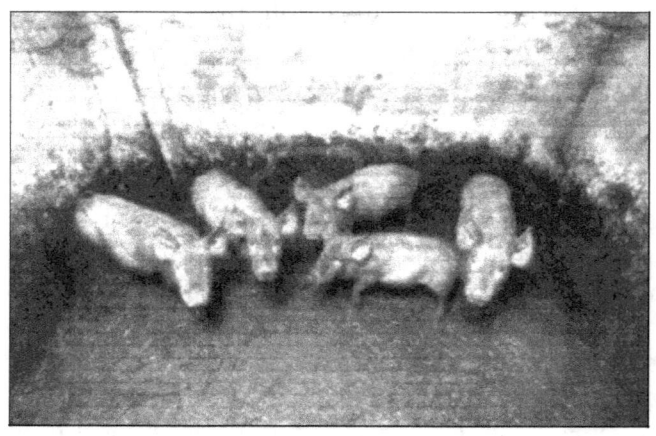

Would you like a pork chop?

Let me concur with Dr. Albert Einstein; —I have no particular talent, I am merely inquisitive.‖ The author.

By the author

My sole motivation with these writings is to convey to my fellow man some of the goodies of a healthy life that I have learned and experienced over eight decades. It is not pleasant to see so many of one's relatives and friends go to their graves at a relatively young age whilst one walks around knowing how death could have been prevented. I give it to you from a Christian perspective in my own self-humble way. If any one should improve this work, may his or her hand be blessed in writing. Information is taken from public domain, and that which I have researched and owe thanks to different institutes. The saying goes —One ounce of prevention is better than a pound of cure‖.

All scientific discoveries are but an elaboration of that which is already fundamentally expressed in the —Maker's Hand Book‖. I know it sounds like a sweeping statement, and yet it is a substantiated claim. WHAT THE BIBLE SAYS ABOUT HEALTHY LIVING is based on three simple principles: 1) Eat the foods God created for you. 2) Don't alter God's design. 3) Don't let any food or drink become your God. Imagine, millennia gone by since the man of YAHWEH wrote a proper hygienic procedure in the Maker's Handbook, and it still works.

The most dangerous enemy is the invisible enemy. It is no superstition to believe in evil demonic forces at work. It is also no superstition to believe that little critters that are of microbe size are perpetually attacking living beings. They are invisible to the naked eye. Never the less, they are very dangerous little microbes.

You may rightfully say to me —get on with it man, don't beat around the bush; tell me the reason for your extended healthy life.‖ In short let me just say that I was raised with the Ten Commandments being drilled into me; especially the one that says —Honor your father and your mother, so that you may have a long life in the land that God gives you.‖ Knowing the —Big Ten,‖ will inevitably cause you to live a clean life, and hygiene is imperative for a healthy life. A news reporter once asked a hundred and three year old lady if she could tell him how she attained a century of good health; her answer was without hesitation —I honored my father and mother and kept God's commandments.‖

Your Creator knows best. It is, therefore, of the greatest importance that we refer to His Book to see what is conducive and what is not good for us as fragile human creatures. The Ten Commandments and the other laws are for our good; given us from a loving Father's Heart and every one of them is a jewel. The Ten Commandments are simply the Almighty commanding us to heed all the statutes and ordinances. That is to say that each and every one of the TEN is the heading of hundreds of sub commands.

One may rightfully ask the question —What could be the cause of this magnificent bunch of molecules to get sick and weary of this

wonderful life on this wonderful creation of nature?‖ And —What is it that causes this body, so wonderfully constructed and certified by its Creator as _Good' to die?‖ The main cause of that misery is SIN. You define SIN by: disobedience to the Law Of the Creator.‖ What law? That which is so clearly spelled out in the Maker's Hand Book called the Bible. Mankind is guilty of breaking God's Laws on a daily basis; yes, even from our first mother who ate of that which Yahshua had said, —But of the tree of the knowledge of good and evil, thou shalt not eat of it: for in the day that thou eatest thereof thou shalt surely die.‖ Now we still eat of that which He forbade His creatures to eat. I know you will find an argument to contravene this one.

The Creator, being the second Person in the Godhead, once told a man in John 5:14, Afterward Yahshua [Jesus] findeth him in the temple, and said unto him, Behold, thou art made whole: sin no more, lest a worse thing befall thee. It is my sincere belief that mankind, as the crown of creation, could live a much healthier life if we quit violating the laws of Elohim YAH. For clarification: Elohim refers to the Trinity. Yah is the Name of the God of the Bible. The word God refers to an object of worship. The God of the Bible says in Psalms 68:4 Sing unto Elohim, sing praises to his name: extol him that rideth upon the heavens by his name YAH, and rejoice before him.

When we say —Halluuw Yah,‖ it simply means —Praise be to

Yahweh.‖ I prefer not to nick name the Almighty. With this work I wish to offer my humble efforts to demonstrate how the wonderful prevention of diseases in the Old Testament compare with modern medical discoveries. Discovery of practices commanded way back as far as three thousand years ago, by that great man of YAHWEH, named Moses. May this book help millions to live a healthier life and may it remind our beloved doctors of some highlights in medical history.

The Word says in Ecclesiastes 1:9. The thing that hath been, it is that which shall be; and that which is done is that which shall be done: and there is no new thing under the sun. 1:10 Is there any thing whereof it may be said, See, this is new? it hath been already of old time, which was before us. Is it not strange that some fossils of excellent tools and boots are found in the same excavated layers as dinosaurs and silocanths. In this volume is found testimonies of natural healings as well as scientific researches done on so many things that can damage our health.

I owe a particular debt of gratitude to Samuel Woodall for his advice and input when spending endless hours proofreading, critique and recommendations. As I have stated, I have no particular talent, but purely relied on them that had gone before me.

I lift my glass to you, dear reader, and wish you a happy and healthy life. —Cheers!‖

The Editor's Comments

In the 1960's, as a young undergraduate student, my favorite biology professor challenged me to independently study the early pioneering scientists of the 17th, 18th, and 19th centuries, to gain an appreciation of their perseverance and diligence in pursuing —pure science‖ and the discoveries that followed. That was his method of encouraging me to —go and do likewise.‖ Cobus van der Merwe has reminded me of that study, but with an important addition. He has brought the Word of God, The Holy Scriptures, to shine its true light on the —discoveries‖ of science and medicine. Our Creator has revealed Himself, in creation and in His Word, to be our loving Father, One who desires only the best
of life for us. But we follow our human father, Adam, in rejecting or questioning His Word and the result is we fall prey to every evil device of the great deceiver—Lucifer, the devil.

Mr. Van der Merwe has compiled historic medical —discoveries‖ and anecdotal accounts that reinforce the ideas and truths concerning human health that were first given as instructions to mankind from the very mind of God. Through this book, may you have the illumination needed to see the errors of following Doubter's Path and, instead, regain and remember the —old paths‖ that lead to a healthy and joyful life in Christ!

What The Docs Say

<u>Dr. O'Roark D.O.:</u> As a third year medical student in 1983, it was increasingly apparent that I wanted to study and eventually practice cardiology. I purchased a copy of J. Willis Hurst's' —The **Heart**", a classic in the field of cardiovascular medicine and read it intensively.

Dr. Hurst was not simply concerned in teaching his students only about current trends in cardiovascular diagnosis and therapy but displayed a tremendous interest in relaying information regarding the history of medicine especially as it pertained to the cardiovascular sciences. Historical vignettes were liberally sprinkled throughout the book. He felt that students of the medical sciences would be well served by a knowledge of what had been done in the past as well as what was known in the present. This knowledge would lay a foundation for a future of lifelong learning and discovery.

Likewise, our author, the esteemed Cobus Van Der Merwe, has emulated the goals of Dr. Hurst and has the lay reader as his target audience. In this concise work, he covers the history behind many seminal events in medical discovery: equipment (stethoscope, thermometer), disease transmission (Walter Reed and mosquitoes, Semmelweis and hand washing) and the importance of healthy eating to name but a few. Where possible, he shows how these tools and discoveries have been used to prevent disease, not merely treat it.

Most importantly, the book takes a holistic view of man as revealed in God's Word, The Bible. The author takes great care in examining the various medical discoveries in the context of Biblical teaching. One is comforted to see, as always, that modern scientific discovery is completely compatible with

Christian teaching and that the teachings of Scripture will never be truly contradicted by any scientific discovery.

Mr. Van Der Merwe is to be commended for his wonderful little book and his ongoing, humble service to Christ his King!

--

Dr. Wyker: I very much enjoyed reading your history of biblical influences on our health and the profession.

I am honored that you would want me to be a part of this fascinating and educational text.

I, however, do not feel comfortable adding to what the Great Physician has already said, nor to the eloquent words already written by the editor.

Your work stands as a high achievement on its own, not requiring any of my words, which I feel would fall short of adequate praise.

Thank you for sharing your work with me.

Arthur Wyker M.D.

—And it was Good.‖ The first Adam.
Consider this magnificent complication and stand in awe

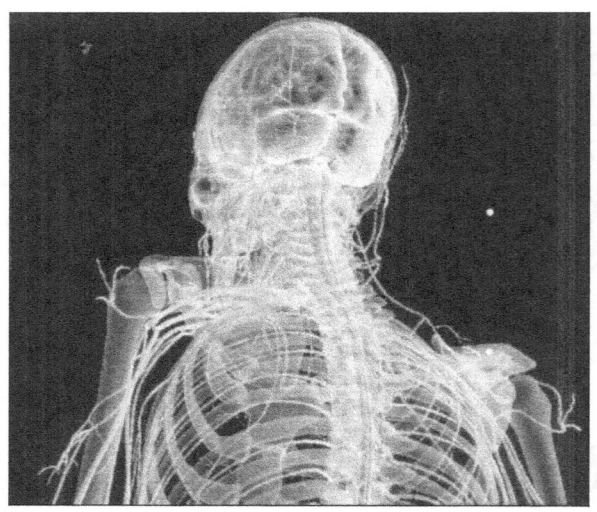

What a design!

Better to hunt in fields for health unbought
Than fee the doctor for a nauseous draught
The wise, for cure, on exercise depend
God never made His work for man to mend.
John Dryden

Doesn't he look pretty cool? Thanks to The late Mr. Fahrenheit you can just poke a sensor in his ear and right away it will tell his coolness, or well on the other hand his temperature to see if he is really as cool as he looks. Fahrenheit is the temperature scale proposed in 1724 by, and named after, the Dutch-German-Polish physicist, Daniel Gabriel Fahrenheit (1686–1736). Today, the temperature scale has been replaced by the Celsius scale in most countries, but it remains the official scale of the United States. Three tools of the trade are indispensable to the doctor, one being the —Fever pin‖ and the other two the blood pressure monitor and stethoscope. The last two mentioned will be dealt with later. I just thought it fit to begin with the thermometer.

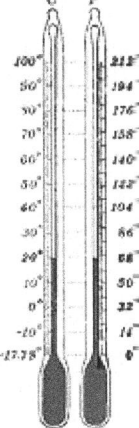

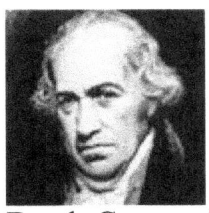

Dutch-German-Polish physicist Daniel Gabriel Fahrenheit (1686–1736)

It was king Solomon that once had said —My son, there is no end in making books‖. One may say the same thing about inventions; the one invention leads to many others. Cobus

ADAM

Man was created a perfect being in every way; the capaciousness of the brain of this super intelligent creature is yet to be established. With all his achievements, man is subjected to all sorts of diseases. Numerous institutes, laboratories, and workplaces packed with learnt people are perpetually busy seeking out the myriad of man's invisible- to- the- naked- eye enemies that are constantly out to destroy him. We are thankful to for providing scientists that devote their lives in search of things that our Creator helps keep man going. That is so; however, we are inclined to neglect some good advice offered to us in the Maker's Handbook. Is it because it is free? More than often people would buy an expensive apparatus that is to be assembled, then get started putting the parts together only to discover that being a smart Alec does not always work out alright. Then in desperation will pick up the maker's handbook and by studying it they discover their mistakes. Only when their mistakes are known, they become real smart.

Benjamin Franklin said, —God heals and the doctor takes the fee.‖

The Dutchman's Glass

By the middle of the seventeenth century, whilst my ancestors under the leadership of Dr. Jan van Riebeeck M.D. were getting settled in the Cape of Good Hope, after three months at sea from Amsterdam, great things were astir in the world. Here and there men were thumbing their noses at almost everything that passed for knowledge. In England, a few of these rebels started a society called The Invisible College--it had to be invisible because Oliver Cromwell might have hanged them for plotters and heretics if he had heard of the strange questions they were trying to settle. One of the members was Robert Boyle, founder of the science of chemistry, and another was Isaac Newton. When Charles II came to the throne, this college became the Royal Society of England. And it was Anton van Leeuwenhoek's first   audience.

Antonie Philips van Leeuwenhoek (in Dutch also Anthonie, Antoni, or Theunis and In English, Anthony or Anton) born on October 24, 1632 – baptized on November 4. His family name Anglicized would be —Lions corner.‖ Leeuwenhoek was a quiet storekeeper with minimal education who made his humble contribution to medical science when he spent his off time on polishing glasses.   He had his little workshop in his house. This Hollander was infatuated with the glass. He would spend hours grinding and shaping glasses. Some convex and some concaved. People thought that he was out of his mind. He discovered that with his convex glasses he could enlarge objects. . Little is known of Leeuwenhoek's early life. When his stepfather died in 1648, he was sent to Amsterdam to become an apprentice to a linen draper. Returning to Delft when he was 20, he established himself as a draper and haberdasher. In

1660 he obtained a position as chamberlain to the sheriffs of Delft. His income was thus secure and sufficient enough to enable him to devote much of his time to his all-absorbing hobby, that of grinding lenses and using them to study tiny objects. Leeuwenhoek made microscopes consisting of a single, high-quality lens of very short focal length; at the time, such simple microscopes were preferable to the compound microscope, which increased the problem of chromatic aberration. Although Leeuwenhoek's studies lacked the organization of formal scientific research, his powers of careful observation enabled him to make discoveries of fundamental importance. In 1674 he began to observe bacteria and protozoa, his "very little animalcules," which he was able to isolate from different sources, such as rainwater, pond and well water, and the human mouth and intestine, and he calculated their sizes.

In 1677 he described for the first time the spermatozoa from insects, dogs, and man, though Stephen Hamm probably was a co-discoverer. Leeuwenhoek studied the structure of the optic lens, striations in muscles, the mouthparts of insects, and the fine structure of plants and discovered parthenogenesis in aphids. In 1680 he noticed that yeasts consist of minute globular particles. He extended Marcello Malpighi's demonstration in 1660 of the blood capillaries by giving (in 1684) the first accurate description of red blood cells. In his observations on rotifers in 1702, Leeuwenhoek remarked that "in all falling rain, carried from gutters into water-butts, animalcules are to be found; and that in all kinds of water, standing in the open air, animalcules can turn up. For these animalcules can be carried over by the wind, along with the bits of dust floating in the air."

One man in Delft did not laugh at Anton van Leeuwenhoek: Reinier de Graaf, a scientist who corresponded with the Royal Society of England. Although Mr. Leeuwenhoek kept all his inventions in magnification secret, he somehow took a liking to Graaff and showed him his magic lenses. What he saw intrigued him so much that he wrote to the Society asking them to persuade Anton to —Write to you telling his discoveries.‖ Leeuwenhoek, from 1673 until 1723, communicated with the Royal Society, by means of informal letters, most of his discoveries. Elected as a Fellow in 1680, his discoveries were, for the most part, made public in the society's Philosophical Transactions. The first representation of bacteria is to be found in a drawing by Leeuwenhoek in that publication in 1683.

His researches on the life histories of various low forms of animal life were in opposition to the doctrine that they could be produced spontaneously or bred from corruption. Thus, he showed that the weevils of granaries (in his time commonly supposed to be bred from wheat as well as in it) are really grubs hatched from eggs deposited by winged insects. His letter on the flea, in which he not only described its structure, but traced out the whole history of its metamorphosis, is of great interest, not so much for the exactness of his observations as for an illustration of his opposition to the spontaneous generation of many lower organisms, such as "this minute and despised creature." Some theorists asserted that the flea was produced from sand, others from dust or the like, but Leeuwenhoek proved that it bred in the regular way of winged insects.

Leeuwenhoek, also, carefully studied the history of the ant and was the first to show that what had been commonly reputed to be ants' eggs were really their pupae, containing the perfect insect nearly ready for emergence, and that the true eggs were much smaller and gave origin to maggots, or larvae. He argued that the sea mussel and other shellfish were not generated out of sand found at the seashore or mud in the beds of rivers at low water but from spawn, by the regular course of generation. He maintained the same to be true of the freshwater mussel, whose embryos he examined so carefully that he was able to observe how they were consumed by "animalcules," many of which, according to his description, must have included ciliates in conjugation, flagellates, and the Vorticella. Similarly, he investigated the generation of eels, which were at that time supposed to be produced from dew without the ordinary process of generation.

The dramatic nature of his discoveries made him world famous, and he was visited by many notables--including Peter I the Great of Russia, James II of England, and Frederick II the Great of Prussia.

Leeuwenhoek's methods of microscopy, which he kept secret, remain something of a mystery. During his lifetime he ground more than 400 lenses, most of which were very small--some no larger than a pinhead--and usually mounted them between two thin brass plates, riveted together. A large sample of these lenses, bequeathed to the Royal Society, were found to have magnifying powers of between 50 and, at the most, 300 times. In order to observe phenomena as small as bacteria, Leeuwenhoek must have employed some form of oblique illumination, or other technique, for enhancing the effectiveness of the lens, but this method he would not reveal. Leeuwenhoek continued his work almost to the end of his long life of 90 years. We as human beings owe a lot to that —Uneducated‖ great scientist Anton Leeuwenhoek for the microscope, an indispensable instrument in the medical world. We will look at just a few of the many microscopic discoveries under the lens of Mijn Heer van Leeuwenhoek's microscope. Most of modern day discoveries are mere rediscoveries of that what was known for as long as thousands of years ago. As we go along we will see the various rediscoveries comparing it with Scripture. The —Truth‖ is a wonderful thing that endureth forever. It is a precious thing and should always be desired. Truth is eternal but Lies need to be invented.

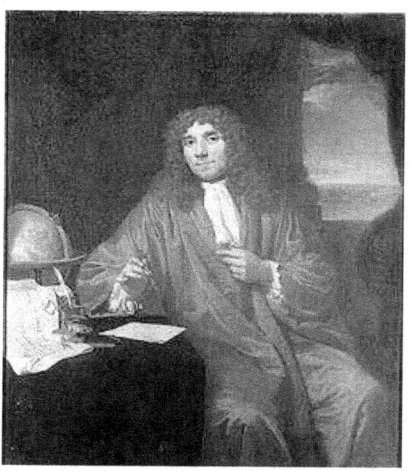

Antonie van **Leeuwenhoek** (1632–1723 By Jan verkolje.

Bed Fever, —The Mother Killer‖

What a wonderful period the nineteenth century must have been. So many great men appeared on the world scene. Not only in the medical field but also in general industry. For example, that century gave us the telephone inventor Alexander Graham Bell and the telegraph inventor Samuel Morse. Radio owes its development to the mentioned two inventions although it only appeared in 1927. In the same glorious century came motorized transportation by Carl Benz. It was as if the population of the globe became impatient with the status quo. There was such a need for better medication and transportation etc. It just seemed that more and more people were dying. Well, there was a population explosion, and the more people are born the more people die. As the saying goes, —There are only two sure things, namely taxes and death.‖ Ronald Reagan said, —We all have a rendezvous with death.‖

I remember vividly the day when my playmate in fifth grade, Dirk Booysen came to school with eyes filled with tears and shared with the class the tragedy that befell their family; his mother died but the baby was saved. As children, the details were kept from us. I could sympathize with my little friend because it was only a year prior that my mother was taken from us as a result of a murderous servant. Losing one's mother, especially at that young age, is something that you never overcome. It was bed fever that killed Mrs. Booysen.

When mamma called, —Come on children, wash your hands and come, eat.‖ Was mother concerned about us messing up the tablecloth? Or was she concerned about our welfare. Mother knows about the germs clinging to our hands; microbes of different strands that quite often cause the death of people.

Great scientists had offered up their lives to prove a very important discovery, of the behavior of microbes. Thanks again to Leeuwenhoek for his devoted hard labor.

We will now take for an example a once despised doctor who proved that animalcules could hide under the skin.

 Whilst thousands of mothers were dying at childbirth, Dr. Ignaz Semmelweis [Born to Jewish parents in 1818 in Ofen, Hungary] was ridiculed by medical science when he discovered the critical importance of the washing of hands by medical professionals in running water and not in a tub, for washing in a basin you merely recycle the microbes. Despite all his efforts to show the medical world how the fatality rate dropped to zero where he was in charge of the Austrian Hospital maternity wards, by simply having his staff wash their hands in running water scrubbing under the tap. Dr Semmelweis had a long battle o v e r many years. It was professional jealousy on the part of the medical hierarchy.

With the help of his microscopes, asserted that in semen of all male animals there were a number of animal-culae in each of which were contained the perfect rudiments of a future animal of the same kind.‖ This discovery of Leeuenhoek was something that gave Dr. Semmelweis much to think about. He repeated, —Microscopic living creatures can hide under the scales of the skin.‖

He was elated one day when he received an encouraging letter from Dr. Kugelmann of Hanover, a former student of the great Professor Michaelis: —Permit me to express the holy joy with which I read your work to a colleague I felt compelled to declare: This man is another Jenner. It has been vouchsafed to very few to confer great and permanent upon mankind, and with few exceptions the world has crucified and burned its benefactors of which our Savior happened to be the greatest of them all. I hope sir doctor you will not grow weary in the honorable fight, which still remains before you.‘‖

Ignaz‘s discovery was publicized worldwide. With the letter had come a parcel; beneath the wrapping were a book and a sheet of paper. On it was written: I humbly beg of you to accept my gratitude in my most prized possession. He opened the book. It was the first edition of Jenner‘s original work, autographed by Jenner himself.

The Etiology had gone out into the entire world. He read, and the little space of hope he had, vanished in a second. The great Virchow, the man to whom all the world of medicine looked with reverence, rose at the German Society For The Advancement of Natural and Medical Sciences and said coldly that childbed fever was caused by erysipelas and inflammation of the lymph glands. Then wise guy Doctor Hecker of Munich proclaimed indignantly:
—The strictest of cleanliness is of little use in preventing such colossal outbreaks of childbed fever as we experience here. The doctrine of Doctor Semmelweis is one-sided, and narrow and erroneous.

Ignaz Philip Semmelweis, a middle-aged old man, stooped and sad, made a final decision to do as His Savior once said that the greatest love is for someone to lay down his life for his friends: the now infamous doctor, for the last time kissed his wife and children goodbye and walked to the hospital. This was not his place of work, but he went straight to the theatre where a cadaver was lying; he sliced his hand and put it in the uterus of the deceased woman; death had not to wait too long to take this, now a devout Christian. The autopsy, done by a famous surgeon showed that the cause of death was —Child bed fever.

In 1890, not withstanding the strenuous protests of Austria and Germany, where it was now claimed that Dr. Semmelweis was a German. Why did they not give the flowers when he was alive? The doctor's Hungarian mother, now conscious of her great son, took his body from Vienna to Budapest for burial in a Church court. In 1906 a statue was unveiled in his honor in the city of his birth. In the world today puerperal fever has by no means disappeared. Yet the children and the mothers his doctrine saved, the great men and women who live because he died are as countless and unimaginable as the sand on the seashore. His beloved daughter Antonia was married in 1882 and bore two sons and two daughters. His beloved Maria lived past the turn of the century with her daughter Margit. His son Bela, who worshipped his father with a silent and utter intensity, grieved for years after his death, and, despairing that his father's teachings would ever be accepted, killed himself at the age of twenty-five.

SIR WILLIAM SINCLAIR, 1909 Professor of Gynaecology and Obstetrics University of Manchester wrote: It is the doctrine of Semmelweis, which lies at the foundation of all our practical work of today. Through all the details of prevention and treatment, the temporary fashions and the changes of nomenclature, the principles of Semmelweis have remained our steadfast guide. The great revolution of modern times in Obstetrics as well as in Surgery is the result of the one idea that, complete and clear, first arose in the mind of Semmelweis, and was embodied in the practice of which he was the pioneer.

—Without Semmelweis my achievements would be nothing.
To this great son of Hungary Surgery owes most.‖

Joseph, Lord Lister, 1906 Professor of Surgery King's College, London, —The beginning was with God. And the end, also.‖

Now today, when a surgeon prepares for an operation he turns on the faucet and scrubs his hands for about ten minutes under the tap. Why does he not just wash his hands in a bowl? Because, thanks to Dr. Semmelweis who gave his own life to prove that germs hide under the scales of the skin, and are carried to the body of the patient by hands. Thus by washing in a basin you merely re-circulate the germs.

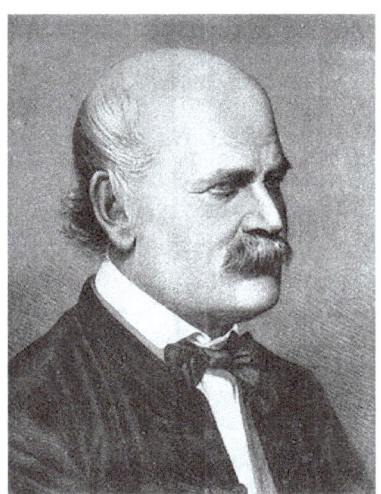

A pen drawing by Miss Semmelweis of her father,

August 13 1865 Ignaz Semmelweis passed on to his abode in Paradise, but only after having given his life for saving the lives of millions of mothers.

The Maker's Handbook:

Mozes in circa 1600 BC led over 2,000,000 people out of Egypt through a barren desert; and I read not of one child lost by childbirth. You see the Maker of the human body provided the Chosen Race with the —Makers Handbook‖ telling them what to do to stay healthy. But as time marched on, mankind seemed to have followed their man made wisdom.

Today we know, since the discovery of bacteriology that many diseases are caused by microorganisms called —bacteria‖ or

—germs‖. In prevention of disease we must isolate or quarantine those who are affected and spread the germs. In a further chapter we will consider the discoverers of these dangerous microbes. For now let us see what the Bible tells about them as far back as 3500 years ago.

Ye shall know the truth and the truth shall make you free. John 8:32.

Quarantine:

I just had to giggle when searching the history books in research for records on the earliest practice of segregating people with contagious diseases to prevent spreading and I came upon this passage: The first known law of segregation on account of disease was enacted by the Emperor Justinian in AD 542. The earliest definite regulations against the spread of disease were, however, developed by Italian city-states under the threat of bubonic plague in the fourteenth century. Venice, the great entrepôt of trade with the east, probably issued regulations as early as 1127, and was the first city to issue a complete quarantine code in 1448. This code provided the model for all subsequent regulations over the next four centuries. Initially these European quarantines were limited to the exclusion of goods and people from stricken localities, but as time went on they were increasingly extended to foreign places as well, especially in seaports.

According to the Bible, during the exodus 1700 B.C. the Israelites with leprosy or other communicable diseases were isolated outside the camp away from all others. Leviticus 13:46 all the days wherein the plague shall be in him he shall be defiled; he is unclean: he shall dwell alone; without the camp shall his habitation be. Leviticus 14: This shall be the law of the leper in the day of his cleansing: He shall be brought unto the priest: 3. And the priest shall go forth out of the camp; and the priest shall look, and, behold, if the plague of leprosy were healed in the leper;

4. Then shall the priest command to take for him that is to be cleansed two birds alive and clean, and cedar wood, and scarlet, and hyssop:

5. And the priest shall command that one of the birds be killed in an earthen vessel over running water: When they had been healed they were declared clean by the priest, God's physician, and after thorough washing of the patient and all that had touched was to be burned with fire or sterilized by fire. The saddle he rode on et al, the clothing he wore and the vessel he used and in

some cases even the house were destroyed. Yes, Moses knew his bacteriology. We have only known it since days of Louis Pasteur and Koch and the microscope of Leeuwenhoek, only because of our ignorance of the Maker's handbook.

Have you ever watched a surgeon preparing for an operation? If you have, you noticed that he goes to the faucet, turns it on and then scrubs his hands for from ten to fifteen minutes under the running tap. Why does he not wash in a bowl? Because infection is carried over to the body by hands where these germs hide under the scales of the skin. The moment the physician, therefore, touches the water in the bowl the water becomes contaminated, and no matter how long he washes in that disease-laden water, his hands can never be rid of the germs. So he puts them under the tap and scrubs them, loosening the scales of skin tissue and the germs, which are carried away by the running water, till his hands are "surgically clean" and he can handle his patient without danger of infection.

Moses knew all that 3,500 years before Pasteur was born. Read Leviticus 15 if you want an ultra-scientific discussion of the Biblical rules for disinfection of contagious disease. We read from the thirteenth verse, which deals with the disinfection of the body of a man who had been infected: And when he that hath an issue is cleansed of his issue; then he shall number to himself seven days for his cleansing, and wash his clothes, and bathe his flesh in running water, and shall be clean [Leviticus 15:13].

The Messiah's Word, when He refers to —Nothing that goes into

your mouth will make you unclean‖ is again taken out of context. He knew that the Jews were eating kosher food. He was referring to what came out of the mouth. In other words, the words you use to damage your fellow man; that could make you unclean. The Master was referring to the spiritual man.

Why do we call attention to these things? Because we are living in a day and age when it is considered "smart" to doubt the Word of God. Those who still believe in the infallibility of the Bible are considered old-fashioned. What a shame on the human race having yielded to Satan.

I am not trying to defend the Word of the living God for it stands on its own legs and has been standing for thousands of years;

Yes, not only since Mozes but since creation. The Bible will be opened in judgment day that is for sure.

My question remains: why would we not, I mean at least the Christian people, read the ―Makers handbook? If you ask me, and yes, I think I know, it is because we think we are ―Smart.‖

So, who was EDWARD JENNER? 1800s AD

It was the great Professor Michaelis, remember, who called Dr. Ignaz Semmelweis a second Jenner. Dr. Edward Jenner was an English country doctor who pioneered vaccination. Jenner's discovery in 1796 that inoculation with cowpox gave immunity to smallpox was an immense medical breakthrough and has saved countless lives. In the old days you found medical doctors were divided in three categories viz: country doctor, town doctor and surgeon. Each required special training and stiff examinations. My wife's great grandfather, Dr. Mozes Judah Rood M.D., a Dutch/South African surgeon, was summoned to appear before an examination board in The Hague for prescribing internal medicine whilst he was yet awaiting the issuance of his country doctor certification, and that after he had successfully written his exam. Dr. Rood was a contemporary of Dr. Semmelweis. His final resting place is in the Dutch Reform Church cemetery in Malmesbury South Africa. This old doctor literally worked himself to death during a flu epidemic; yes, day and night without sleep.

Edward Jenner was born on May 17 1749 in the small village of Berkeley in Gloucestershire. From an early age Jenner was a keen observer of nature and after nine years as a surgeon's apprentice he went to St George's Hospital, London to study anatomy and surgery under the prominent surgeon John Hunter. After completing his studies, he returned to Berkeley to set up a medical practice where he stayed until his death in 1823.

EDWARD JENNER SMALLPOX VACCINATION?

Physicians of yesteryear were called on for not only mankind but also for animal kind. Jenner worked in a rural community and most of his patients were farmers or worked on farms with cattle. Small pox in the 18th century was a very common disease and was a major cause of death. The main treatment was by a method, which had brought success to a Dutch physiologist Jan Ingenhaus and was brought to England in 1721 from Turkey by Lady Mary Wortly Montague. This method involved inoculating healthy people with substances from the pustules of those who had a mild case of the disease, but this often had fatal results.

In 1788 an epidemic of smallpox hit Gloucestershire and during this outbreak Jenner observed that those of his patients who worked with cattle and had come in contact with the much milder disease called —Cow pox‖ never came down with smallpox. Jenner needed a way of showing that his theory actually worked. Jenner was given the opportunity on the 14th May 1796, when a young milkmaid called Sarah Nelmes came to see him with sores on her hands like blisters. Jenner identified that she had caught cowpox from the cows she handled each day.

Jenner now had the opportunity to obtain the material to try out his theories. He carefully extracted some liquid from her sores and then took some liquid from the sores of a patient with mild smallpox.

Jenner believed that if he could inject someone with cowpox, the germs from the cowpox would make the body able to defend itself against the dangerous smallpox-germs, which he would inject later.

Jenner approached a local farmer called Phipps and asked him if he could inoculate his son James against smallpox. He explained to the farmer that if his theory were correct, James would never contract smallpox. Surprisingly, the farmer agreed.

Jenner made two small cuts on James's left arm. He then poured the liquid from Sarah's cowpox sores into the open wounds, which he bandaged. I remember as a six-year-old child, I was inoculated the same way; the nurse made scratches on my left arm, about like a quarter in size, one inch in diameter and smeared the vaccine onto the area. Now at the age of 84, the two scars are still visible and whenever I visit a doctor's office for a painless thin needle flu shot, I show off my lesions with pride.

James went down with cowpox but was not very ill. Six weeks later when James had recovered, Jenner vaccinated him again, this time with the smallpox virus.

This was an extremely dangerous experiment. If James lived, Jenner would have found a way of preventing smallpox. If James developed smallpox and died, he would be a murderer.

To Jenner's relief James did not catch smallpox. His experiment had worked.

In 1798 after carrying out further successful tests, he published his findings: An Inquiry into the Causes and Effects of the Variolae Vaccinae, a Disease Known by the Name of Cow Pox. Jenner called his idea "vaccination" from the word vaccinia, which is Latin for cowpox. Jenner also introduced the term virus.

Jenner found a great deal of skepticism to his ideas and was subject to much ridicule. A cartoon was drawn, showing cows coming out of various parts of people's bodies after they had been vaccinated with cowpox.

However, Jenner persevered and eventually, doctors found that vaccination did work and by 1800 most were using it. Jenner was awarded £30,000 by Parliament to enable him to continue carrying out his tests. Deaths from smallpox plummeted and vaccination spread through Europe, South Africa, Australia and North America.

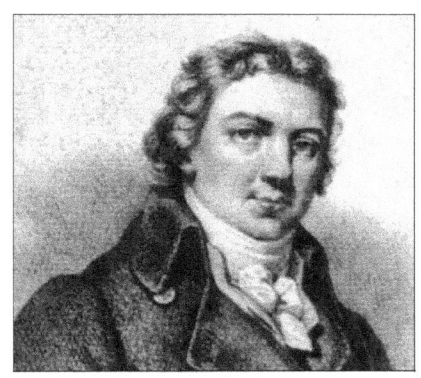

Edward Jenner
Jenner died in Berkeley on January 26, 1823 aged 74. We honor
him in memory, and thank God for giving us men like him.

The Confluence of Many Streams 1800s

President Ronald Reagan gave an oration at one of our elite universities where he was interrupted by a young student —Mr. President‖ he says —You are of the old school; we are of the time of the computers and jet planes.‖ The old president smiled, rubbed his nose and said —Well, that may be so; but, we invented them for you.‖

During the nineteenth century a myriad of inventions surprised the world. It is the century that gave us the first automobile by Carl Benz 1885, the electric light by Thomas Alva Edison, one of the everyday conveniences that most affects our lives, was invented in 1879 by Thomas Alva Edison. He put together what he knew about electricity with what he knew about gaslights and invented a whole electrical system. . It is without question the era that marks the most phenomenal progress in medical history. As we have said, the one invention led to the other like rivulets flowing from different areas into one great stream. There was the man that gave us the Radio in 1927, seneor Marconi of Bologna in Italy, son of an Italian farmer and an Irish mother. I paid a visit to that home many years later. Even he scraped together bits and pieces of what he learned from others like engineer Hertz in Germany who discovered for us the radio waves. Heinrich Rudolf Hertz (February 22, 1857 – January 1, 1894) was a German physicist who clarified and expanded the electromagnetic theory of light that had been put forth by Maxwell. He was the first to satisfactorily demonstrate the existence of electromagnetic waves by building an apparatus to produce and detect VHF or UHF radio waves. So, you can see that all great inventers had common sense to put two and two together.

Leeuenhoek invented for us the microscope for the doctor to see, Edison invented the light without which doctor cannot see that microbe and Marconi invented for us the radio and Hertz the wave, without which we would not have x-ray machines. OK, now you will ask what the motorcar has to do with the above? For one, to get you to the doctor quickly.

The Bible says, —I told you so‖ as we see in the last chapter of Daniel the prophet Daniel 12:10   Many shall purify themselves, and make themselves white, and be refined; but the wicked shall do wickedly; and none of the wicked shall understand; but they that are wise shall understand.

A young lass, named Tossy and her parents, real city slickers, paid us a visit on the farm Excelsior. As boys we did not tolerate girls around us. It happened so that this lassie was a bit of a nuisance to us and insisted to accompany us around the farm. I love a glass of cold milk; in fact, growing up on a farm, my younger brother and I were regular visitors at the corral by cow-milking time; that is to say circa sunset. Armored with our mugs and a slice of fresh baked bread warm out of the brick oven, we got our mugs filled with that foamy milk, still warm from the cow's udder. Then when this little city girl saw where the milk came from, she ran back to the house and never put her lips to milk again. She also quit following us boys around. We, Steve and I, are now well in our eighties and are blessed with having strong bone structures and I even still enjoy my full set of God given teeth.

Looking at the milk container you read the word "Pasteurized", it is so named after the doctor that first discovered the microbes in milk, and came up with an effective way of rendering harmless any disease germs it may contain, particularly tubercle bacilli. The milk is kept for half an hour at a heat of 145-150 degrees Fahrenheit and then cooled. In some countries pasteurization was enforced by law before milk could be sold. Now, other methods are applied, like running the milk over ice.

I recall a health care lesson we had in standard three; [equal to American fifth grade] the teacher, Mr. Nico Swart told us about the importance of pasteurizing the milk ere we drink it. He told us a most intriguing story of the discovery of germs in milk that can kill you. — He went on: —One day, at the Academy of Medicine in Paris, a famous physician was giving an oration, with plenty of long Greek and Latin words, on the cause alas, completely unknown to him of childbed fever. Suddenly he was interrupted by a bellow from the rear of the hall: "The thing that kills women with childbed fever isn't anything like that! It is you doctors who carry deadly microbes from sick women to healthy ones!" It was Louis Pasteur who said this; he was out of his seat; his eyes flamed with excitement.

"Possibly you are right, but I fear you will never find that microbe" By this time Pasteur was charging up the aisle, his left leg, partly paralyzed from a stroke, dragging a little. He reached the blackboard, grabbed a piece of chalk and shouted: "You say I will not find the microbe? I have found it; here's the way it looks!" Louis Pasteur scrawled a chain of little circles on the blackboard. The meeting broke up in confusion.

Pasteur was in his late fifties at this time, but he was still as impetuous and enthusiastic as he had been at twenty-five. The son of a tanner of Arbois, he had become a kind of assistant teacher at the college of Besançon before he was twenty. His father sent him to Paris to the Normal School and there, one day, he discovered the fascination of chemistry. At twenty-six he made his first great discovery: that there is a variety of strange chemical compounds in Nature that are exactly alike, except that they are exact images of each other.

Louis became important overnight and all of a sudden he found himself companion of learned men three times his age. He was appointed a professor at Strasbourg. Where he fell in love and determined to marry the daughter of the dean. He didn't know if she cared for him, but he sat down and wrote her a letter that he would like a way to make her love him: "There is nothing in me to attract a young girl's fancy," he wrote, "but my recollections tell me that those who have known me very well have loved me very much."

So, the daughter of the dean did marry this cripple and became one of the most famous and longsuffering and in many ways one of the happiest wives in history. In the words of Roux, she "loved him even to the point of understanding his work." On those evenings when she was waiting for him, and had finished putting to bed those children, whose absentminded father he was, this brave lady sat primly at a little table and wrote scientific papers at his dictation. Louis was her life. I cannot help but here credit my own daughter in Law Louise, wife of Dr. Andre that stood by him during his student years and did his typing, quite often into the early hours of the morning.

As a viticulturist I am always intrigued reading about his expertise on fermentation. Pasteur showed the French vintners how to keep their wines from spoiling; he saved the sick silkworms of France; he improved French beer. But while he was doing the lifework of a dozen men he dreamed about tracking down the microbes that he knew must be the authors of human disease. He found Koch had done the trick ahead of him. He must catch up with Koch. But there were difficulties in his way. However, he was like a bulldog that just did not retreat; he kept working day and night, growing microbes and then one day he observed that a culture of anthrax bacilli were swarming with contaminating microbes from the air. The following morning there were no anthrax germs left at all; they had been completely choked out by the others. Pasteur jumped to a fine idea: "If the harmless microbes choke out the anthrax bacilli in the bottle, they will do it in the body too!"

At once he tried the fantastic experiment of giving guinea-pigs anthrax and then shooting millions of harmless microbes into them-germs which were to chase the anthrax bacilli round the body and devour them. Pasteur gravely announced: "There are high hopes for the cure of disease from this experiment," but that is the last you hear of it, for he never gave science the benefit of studying his failures. But a little later the Academy of Sciences sent him on a queer errand, and on this mission he stumbled across the first clue to a remarkable way of turning savage microbes into friendly ones.

At this time there was a great to-do about a cure for anthrax invented by a veterinary surgeon, Louvrier, in the Jura Mountains in eastern France. Louvrier had cured hundreds of cows that were at death's door, said the influential men of the district; it was time that this treatment received scientific approval. Pasteur went there, with his young assistants, and found that the miraculous "cure" consisted, first, in getting several farmhands to rub the sick cow violently to make her hot; then long gashes were cut in the poor beast's skin and into these cuts Louvrier poured turpentine; finally the now bellowing cow was covered with a thick layer of unmentionable stuff soaked in hot vinegar. This was kept, by a cloth, on the animal--which doubtless wished she were dead.

Pasteur suggested to Louvrier that they make an experiment. So four healthy cows were brought and Pasteur, in the presence of Louvrier and a solemn commission of farmers, shot a powerful dose of anthrax microbes into the shoulder of each beast. Next day all the cows had large feverish swellings on their shoulders, their breath came in snorts--they were in a bad way.

"Now, Doctor," said Pasteur, "choose two of these sick cows, and give them your cure; and we'll leave the other two without any treatment at all." The result was a terrible blow to the would-be curer of cows, for one of the cows that Louvrier treated got better but the other perished; and one of the creatures that had got no treatment at all, died but the other got better.

So there were two cows left over from the experiment, beasts that had had a siege of anthrax and had recovered. "What shall I do with them?" pondered Pasteur. "Well, I might try shooting a still more savage strain of anthrax into them. I have one family of anthrax germs that would give even a rhinoceros a bad night."

So Pasteur injected his vicious germs into the two cows that had got better. He waited, but the cows remained healthy and happy! So Pasteur jumped to one of his quick conclusions: "Once a cow has survived anthrax, all the anthrax microbes in the world cannot give her another attack.‖

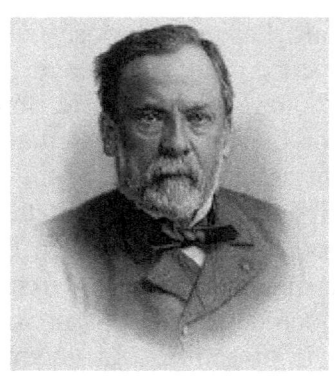

Louis Pasteur

In memoriam we honor this great man lent to us by the Creator.

It was in 1952 that I got to know about old Doc. Crockery of the town of Warmbaths. He was a real old family doctor with unique bedside manners, and very germ conscious. It was during the great flu epidemic that doctor Crockery worked day and night, visiting his patients. One old fellow that remembered the doc's visit to his house, told me the story about how the old man of medicine never entered any home, but cast his long tube stethoscope through the window, then gave directions to an insider as to where to hold the scope. Being then satisfied that he had made the correct diagnosis, gave them a bottle of Bayer's aspirin, and with that his treatment was completed.

Quote by Louis Pasteur: Where observation is concerned, chance favors only the prepared mind.
Contemporary with this godly man were many of the ungodly that called themselves scientists, doing their level best to disprove an Almighty God. Some of them such as Russell devoted their lives to spiritism. Remarkable how many have the name Charles, amongst whom the most known Charles Darwin, Charles Lyell, and the artist Charles Knight etc. On the other hand it seems that they by name —Louis‖ leaned more to the right.
Whilst it was fashionable for someone to be an evolutionist and the talk of the town, Pasteur was a devout Roman Catholic and had been opposed to the idea of spontaneous generation ever

since he had first learned of it. It seemed to him that it was going beyond the biblical dictum that creation of life was a divine operation that had been confined to and completed in the first week of Creation. Then again, Pasteur lost no time in making this clear in writing and in speeches. For example, he wrote in 1864:

To bring about spontaneous generation would be to create a germ. It would be creating life; it would be to solve the problem of its origin. It would mean to go from matter to life through conditions of environment and of matter [non-life]. God as author of life would then no longer be needed. Matter would replace Him. God would need to be invoked only as author of the motions of the universe (Dubois 1976, 395).

Elegantly simple, Pasteur's work won him the coveted French Academy of Science's prize. He well recognized, however, that he had not proven that spontaneous generation did not occur by every imagined means, but he had grandly exposed the fallacy of all previous claims. Nevertheless, the fact that this work was published just two years after Darwin's Origin was particularly damaging to the fledgling theory of evolution for which the spontaneous generation of life from non-life was crucial.

Now may I say, —Dear Dr. Louis, where I grew up were a great variety of apes whom I got to know very well; in fact, they were my friends; thus I know apes when I see them, and I concur with you doctor, those monkeys are no apes.‖

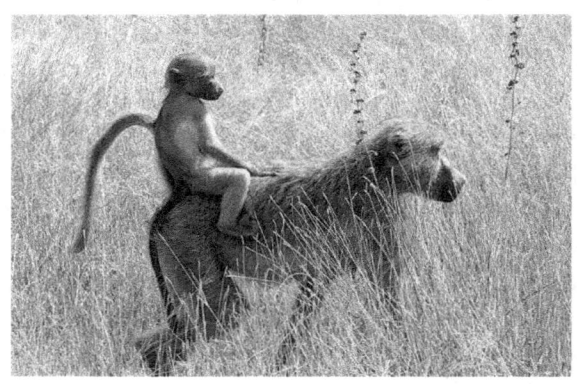

Even though an ape wears a golden ring
He still remains an ugly thing. Cobus

The fear of God is the beginning of wisdom
To learn from your elders
Is to put wisdom at work Cobus

Penicillin weapon against the unseen enemy

One cannot but admire our soldiers fighting terrorists in the Moslem world. Our men have to distinguish the difference between the ordinary man in the street and the almost unidentifiable enemy in civic clothes We may say that our soldiers have the undesirable task of fighting an unseen enemy, very much like our doctors have to fight unseen enemies. Fighting the microbes, the unseen enemies. It would be most unfair so as not to mention the name of a great man that invented a very successful weapon against man's unseen enemy viz, the different microbes. When the white blood cells, the body's soldiers are struggling hard to fight infection and the battle results in high fever it welcomes the help of antibiotic ammunition. For this invention much gratitude is owed to Sir Alexander Flemming who invented penicillin.

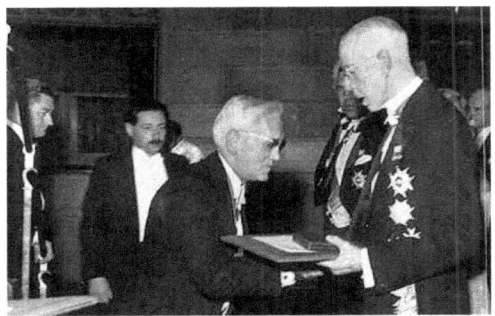

Picture as perWikipedia

Alexander Flemming was born in Lochfield Scotland on August 6, 1881 and passed away on March 11 1955 in London.
Fleming in the center receiving the Nobel Prize from King Gustav V of Sweden in 1945.

Antibiotics

From what I can gather its origin could be ascribed as a starting point. Unfortunately few scientists take the time to record for posterity the course of events which led to the discoveries which were the —fruit of their labor" Dr. Schatz told his own accurate and interesting account of his finding. Streptomycin turned out to be a milestone in the history of drugs to treat tuberculosis and other infections. Dr. Schatz's role has been largely ignored. A New Jersey farmer was upset: his chickens were catching a strange infection from barnyard dirt. He took the birds to the Rutgers University laboratory of microbiologist Selman Waksman, who analyzed the barnyard soil and isolated the problem - a peculiar fungus. In the process, Waksman fortuitously discovered that the microorganism had properties besides the ability to make chickens sick. The fungus produced a chemical agent that slowed the growth of certain bacteria.

Aneasethics

Since the inception of mankind and the fall of our common papa Adam, any incision in our skin caused pain. And looking at history books we find that it often became imperative for surgery to fix from the outside what was wrong in the inside of the body. Most common to almost all people happened to be tonsillectomy and what inevitably followed was appendectomy. The mother of Julius Caesar had to be cut open to remove the stubborn little emperor to be from her abdomen. It happened on the 13th of July 100 B.C. and amazingly, this procedure is still in practice today; just think about it; after two thousand years. This procedure is known as a Caesarian birthǁ or as commonly known in America as simply. —C Sectionǁ.

Watching the old cowboy movies, you often see where they had to, knock the patient out by pistol butt-end. However, this extreme method of anesthetic was only applied when there was nothing stronger, like for instance whiskey, which of course was by far preferred to the pre-mentioned method.

Minor surgeries like a streptococcus- serious infections remedied by streptomycin, an antibiotic drug, related to penicillin, simply had to wait for the preferred Aneasethics made by moonlight. But again, thanks to devoted scientists a better remedy came to mankind, the streptomycin.

I remember the late John Wayne having a slug removed from his seat without a shot of the —holy waterǁ just to prove how tough he was. In fact old John did not believe in drinking just ordinary water; his contention was that water is only used to wash with.

It was one of the great industrialists that once said that to be a millionaire you should find a need, and then fill that need and you're on your way to having it made in the shade. Well, many a fortune seeker has broken his neck to identify a need, but others have just stumbled upon it by chance.

Many thousands of people just took a short cut and kicked the bucket even before the incision was stitched up. Because, pain is pain even from that very first day in the Garden of Eden. I will say a little more about that later.

We as patients take such a lot for granted and quite often have the attitude of —Well I pay them to heal me‖ and that is that; while we do not consider the fact that our doctors have committed their whole lives to sacrifice all, even sometimes their own lives, to keep us above ground.

The medical world was elated when Samuel Guthrie, and David Waldie discovered a breakthrough in Aneasethics. Dr. Sam was not only a physician, but, also, a chemist who devoted his life to pain relief medication. He invented, also, firearm bullet caps that superseded the old musket flintlocks. It was with this invention he became permanently an invalid due to an explosion in prosecuting his experiments in November 1831.

Guthrie wrote of his findings, thus he is generally acknowledged as the discoverer of Chloroform, by distilling chloride of lime with alcohol in a copper barrel. Dr. Sam Guthrie was a son of America, born in Massachusetts in 1782. He was a man of deep faith and a Church member of Congregational Church. One can only guess how many prayers this doctor had prayed for the welfare of his patients. Invariably this kind of person achieves great heights. Scripture tells us that if we acknowledge Him He will direct our paths.

The first very effective Aneasethics was first used by a Doctor Simpson who was the first person to use chloroform as an anesthetic. Dr. James Y. Simpson was born in Bathgate, the seventh son of a baker and went to Edinburgh University at the age of 14. He completed his studies four years later but because of his youth, had to wait another two years before gaining a license to practice medicine. He specialized in obstetrics and became Professor of Midwifery at the University at the age of 28. After experimenting with chloroform on himself and his friends in 1847, he started to use it as an anesthetic to ease the pain of childbirth. Simpson was not the first to use chloroform - Sir Humphrey Davy used Nitrous Oxide (Laughing Gas) in 1799, but it was Simpson's persistent advocacy which led to its acceptance - despite opposition on both medical and religious grounds - it was viewed at the time as "an act against nature or the will of God."

But chloroform was used by Queen Victoria during the birth of Prince Leopold in 1853 and it then gained wide acceptance.

Simpson became the first person to be knighted for services to medicine in 1866. "Victor Dolore" (pain conquered) is the inscription of his coat of arms. When he died in 1870 at the age of 58, an offer of burial in Westminster Abbey in London was declined and instead he was buried at Warriston Cemetery in Edinburgh. 100,000 people turned up for the funeral.

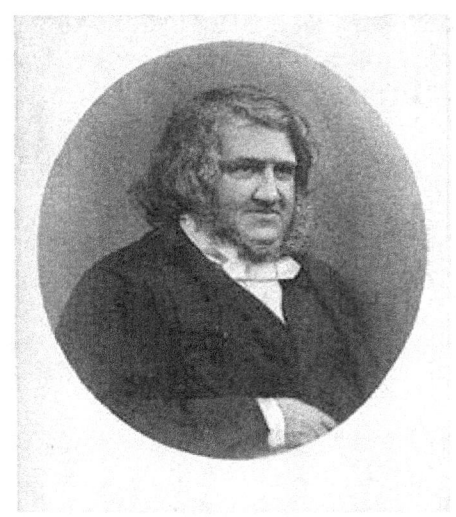

The short and sweet about the first use of Aneasethics and surgery is recorded for us in Genesis 2:21 And Yahweh God caused a deep sleep to fall upon the man, and he slept; and he took one of his ribs, and closed up the flesh instead thereof:

We men were made from clay, but our ladies were made from flesh and bone. This means that we men have little to brag about. And just one more thing; we should always remember that our female counterpart was taken from close to our hearts and not from our foot soles for us trample on, neither from the tops of our heads for them to sit there.

Amazing! People listen to people. Scripture tells us that only a fool believes what he is told, but a wise person checks his way to see where he is going. We've all heard the mockers of the Bible saying, —Ah, until Galileo's discovery, people believed that the earth was flat.‖ True, they were ignorant of the Bible's contents like they are today. Just a few days ago —Old Bozo‖ Albert Gore was saying —Those skeptical folks on the right that don't believe that this globe is steering to complete destruction, also, still believe that the earth is flat.‖ Really?

Galileo Galilei 15 February 1564– 8 January 1642 was an Italian Physicist who played a major role in the Scientific Revolution. His achievements include improvements to the primitive telescope and consequent astronomical observations, and support for Copernicus. Galileo has been called the "father of modern observational astronomy‖, the "father of modern physics, the father of science and the Father of Modern Science. He observed the motion of uniformly accelerated objects, taught in nearly all high school and introductory college physics courses. His contributions to observational astronomy include the telescopic confirmation of the phases of Venus, the discovery of the four largest satellites of Jupiter; named the Galilean moons in his honor, and the observation and analysis of sunspots. Galileo also worked in applied science and technology, improving compass design, which was already a great improvement of the Alkemal. By this period in time of the renaissance, well-meaning people believed that the Earth was central in the universe with all celestial bodies moving around it. They were also of the belief that the Earth was more or less flat.

The Bible had the answer, but like with so many Theologians, even of today, do not really know what Scripture teaches us. I suppose that our figure of speech is sometimes accepted literally; for example, we talk about —Sun-Rise‖ and: "sun-set‖ etc.

Let me just say this: The Bible does not need any of our support; it stands on it's own legs and proves itself correct every time it is being put to the test.

Isaiah 40:21 Have ye not known? have ye not heard? hath it not been told you from the beginning? have ye not understood from the foundation of the earth? 22. It is He that sitteth upon the circle of the earth, and the inhabitants thereof are as grasshoppers; that stretcheth out the heavens as a curtain, and spreadeth them out as a tent to dwell in: Job 38:33 Knowest thou the ordinances of heaven? canst thou set the dominion thereof in the earth? Hello Bozo!

The Messiah Himself talked about in one given moment there shall be midnight, morning and noon, indicating the round earth in movement. This latter quotation refers to the moment of His return. Luke 17:34 I tell you, two people will be in the same bed that night; one will be taken, and the other will be left behind. 35. Two women shall be grinding together [Breakfast]; the one shall be taken, and the other left. Two men shall be in the field [Day]; the one shall be taken, and the other left.

Let me say: True science can never be in conflict with Biblical Scripture. And what's more, the Creator Messiah takes care of His own designed solar system and needs not the help of the godless. What we read in Psalm 2 is so prevalent in our day: Psalms 2:2 The kings of the earth set themselves, and the rulers take counsel together, against the Lord, and against his anointed, saying, `3. Let us break their bands asunder, and cast away their cords from us.

4. He that sitteth in the heavens shall laugh: the Lord shall have them in derision. Yes, they will try at all costs, to you and me, whatever they can to break our bands that bind us to our Savior Messiah God. They will prevent prayer in school; forbid the reading of Scripture; kill the unborn; propagate evolution, and

dish up lies upon lies of which —Global warming‖ is one of the biggies.

Just who do these lefties think they are? They are simply followers of their god, Satan, who has desperately been trying to disprove Almighty God Yahweh since the time of creation.

Psalms 24:1 the earth is Yahweh's, and the fullness thereof; the world, and they that dwell therein. 2 For he hath founded it upon the seas, and established it upon the floods.

Jeremiah 51:15 He hath made the earth by his power, he hath established the world by his wisdom, and by his understanding hath he stretched out the heavens: When he uttereth his voice, there is a multitude of waters in the heavens; and he causeth the vapours to ascend from the ends of the earth: he maketh lightnings with rain, and bringeth forth the wind out of his treasures. Talk about science!

17.   Every man is brutish by his knowledge; every founder is confounded by the graven image: for his molten image is falsehood, and there is no breath in them.

18.   They are vanity, the work of errors: in the time of their visitation they shall perish.   I have heard these Satan's children mocking God's Word by asking ‖On what did God pour his concrete for the earth's foundation?‖ By this question they only prove their ignorance. The answer to those blasphemous creatures is simply Job 26:7 He stretcheth out the north over empty space, And <u>hangeth the earth upon nothing</u>. Now this is solid science. My favorite subject in engineering was magnetic fields, such as the mightiest one sustaining the globe and planets with their satellites.

The Messiah speaks to John in Revelation 5:3 and no one in the heaven, or on the earth, or <u>under the earth</u>, [That is the other side] was able to open the book, or to look thereon.

51

Only a fool says in his heart, —There's no God.‖ Psalms 14: 1. NB. The Almighty God needs no help from man.

University of Scranton Figs' Healing Power

Scranton, PA American Association of Cereal Chemists, Inc.
I quote: J. A. Vinson
University of Scranton

The importance of —nutraceuticals,‖ also known as —functional foods,‖ in the American diet is highlighted by the fact that consumers paid out $9 billion/year for these products (1). The definition of functional foods is still evolving but refers to —foods that, by virtue of physiologically active components, provide benefits beyond basic nutrition and may prevent disease or promote health,‖ as stated by Clare Hasler, director of the University of Illinois Functional Foods for Health Program. Increasingly, manufacturers are including the names of nonnutritive components on their labels. For example, the labels on green tea list —polyphenols,‖ and those on tofu list —isoflavones.‖ The public is becoming more knowledgeable about these nonnutritive ingredients because of the large amount of publicity and articles in the mass media. Today there is an ever-increasing demand for foods that will increase our intake of food components that are perceived to be —protective against disease.‖ In the future, genetic engineering will allow us to provide a variety of fruit or vegetables that is highly elevated in a certain compound. One example of such research is the work by the USDA and others in the development of a tomato high in lycopene, a carotenoid understood to be an antioxidant and anticancer substance. In some varieties, the concentration of lycopene can be three times that of regular tomatoes. The genes responsible for the synthesis of carotenoid such as lycopene have been isolated. The genes have been inserted in an edible yeast and have produced lycopene and Carotenoid at 0.1% dry-weight of isolated cells (2). We are increasingly using foods as preventive agents to decrease our risk of deadly chronic diseases, including cancer and heart disease. The lay person is well aware of the importance of diet to health as a result of the U.S. government's campaign to increase our consumption of fruits and vegetables to five servings/day. This article is designed to provide information on a relatively unknown but extremely —functional‖ fruit, namely figs.

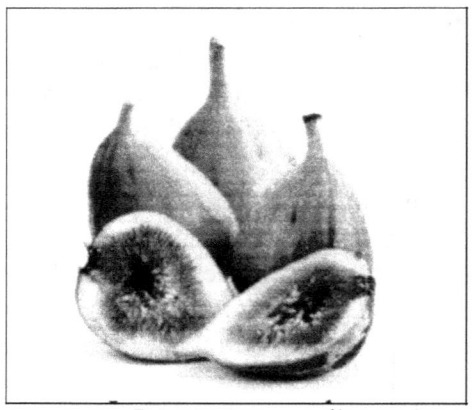
It tastes so good!

[Ficus Carica]   There was a fig tree in the Garden of Eden, and the fig is the most mentioned fruit in the Bible. Genesis 3:7 And the eyes of them both were opened, and they knew that they were naked; and they sewed fig leaves together, and made themselves aprons.

King Hezekiah is certainly one of my favorite kings of the Old Testament and Isaiah was probably one of the greatest of the prophets. When the king was on his deathbed, Yahweh ordered Isaiah to pay him a visit. Isaiah was to inform his majesty that he was going die, and he should make his last will and testament. This great King and civil engineer sought help from the Almighty; he wept and begged his Maker for an extension of his life and Yahweh sent his servant the prophet back to give the king a medicine prescription; 2 Kings 20:77. And Isaiah said, Take a lump of figs. And they took and laid it on the boil, and he recovered. Well, God made man and He surely can fix what so ever goes wrong. I have all reason to believe that this —Boill was not an ordinary boil such as we know it, but a cancer that was about to terminate the king's life

Figs' healing value is only now being rediscovered by the Bible-illiterate world of people. Oh! What a wonderful world this can be if only people would take time and study the Maker's Handbook. In this Greatest Book of science, the fig is mentioned at least fifty times. Even Messiah, when He was hungry sought food from the Fig tree.

So, just read the Maker's handbook and be happy and healthy.

Old Doc. Rosenfeldt answers:

Q. Can increasing potassium intake lower blood pressure?

A. Many studies have shown that increasing dietary potassium intake can lower blood pressure. In addition, there are now several studies, which show that potassium supplementation, al intake alone, can produce significant reductions in blood pressure in hypertensive subjects. Typically these studies have utilized dosages ranging from 2.5 g to 5 g of potassium per day. Significant drops in both systolic and diastolic values have been achieved.
Here is the average K: Na ratios for several common fresh fruits and vegetables:

Carrots: 75:1
Potatoes: ll0: 1
Apples: 99:1
Bananas: 440:1
Oranges: 260:1

A CURE FOR CANCER

Cancer is the Number Two cause of death in the U.S. The use of the product of the vine is widely used by holistic health professionals in other countries to fight disease, often in patients with inoperable cancer. Grapes contain a very powerful antioxidant that protects your body cells from free radicals.

Scientists have given it the name of proanthocyanidins, but it is not new. As far back as 1556, books on this wonderful nature cure had been published in various European languages. The strongest testimony for the grape cure for cancer is a book written by Dr. Johanna Brandt, —The Grape Cure‖ having herself cured from that horrible disease called cancer.

Dr. Brandt was diagnosed with cancer in 1916, shortly after her mother died from cancer. Working with her own diet, fasting, etc., she began to see the relationship of the food she ate to the progression or regression of her cancer. It took nine years to achieve her healing. She discovered that a meat diet perpetuates cancer, a vegetarian diet conquers it, and that organic grapes aid healing. She helped others rid themselves of this deadly disease, left her native South Africa to bring her discovery to the U.S., and wrote this book. She shares her journey back to wellness in this small, yet remarkable book, reprinted because the need is greater than ever for natural discoveries to reach the people.
Grape Juice Can Reverse Memory Loss
Headline story, Friday, December 18, 2009
Oh really? Drinking 100 percent purple grape juice can reduce or even reverse memory loss, according to research by the University of Cincinnati. In a study led by Dr. Robert Krikorian, 12 men and women between the ages of 75 and 80 were divided into two groups. All had been diagnosed with early memory loss. One group drank 100 percent Concord while the other group drank a placebo matched for calories for twelve weeks.

The participants were given memory tests, such as memorizing lists and placing items in a specific order, at regular intervals during the three months. "While there were no significant differences between the groups at baseline, following treatment, those drinking Concord grape juice demonstrated significant improvement in list learning," Krikorian said in a statement. "In addition, trends suggested improved short-term retention and spatial (nonverbal) memory.

"These results with Concord grape juice are very encouraging," he said. "A simple, easy-to-incorporate dietary intervention that could improve or protect memory function, such as drinking Concord grape juice, may be beneficial for the aging population." Other studies have shown that purple grapes have powerful health benefits. One Vanderbilt University study found that people who drank grape juice more than three times a week lowered their risk of developing Alzheimer's by 76 percent.

Additional studies have shown grapes to have heart healthy benefits including keeping arteries supple and blood pressure low. Researchers believe the benefits in Concord grape juice come from antioxidants in the grape's skin and fruit

Oh! This is a great breakthrough in the modern field of medicine. One asks the question —Why only now?‖ grapes have been known to mankind since time immemorial. Let us see if that is really all that new. Let us see what the old Book says about it.

The Healing Power of the Grape
ACCORDING TO MAKER'S HANDBOOK

Once upon a time there was a man named Saul; the name meaning —Requested‖ he was a pious man, a lawyer for that matter. The Bible always formed the foundation of people's constitution; as did the formation of our own constitution that is so despised by the godless left. He knew the —Old Book‖ so well that he developed an obsession in promoting his orthodox faith; so much so that he went all out persecuting them that deviated from what he believed to be the right religion. He especially chased down the followers of the crucified Messiah. One day he was on his way to a little town called Damascus, having with him search/arrest warrants signed and sealed by a high court judge. Meanwhile, the eleven missionaries of the crucified Messiah convened a meeting to elect a replacement of the twelfth apostle named Judas, who betrayed their Master. Their choice was Matthias, a man well known to them; so he was elected to fill that position. Now these apostles were a little forward and did not wait on Messiah to choose His own man for the job, hence the man Matthias never being heard of since. Yahshua the Messiah's choice was the lawyer that was creating havoc among His sheep. He struck him with blindness whilst on his way to Damascus, instructed him to go to a man in Straight Street to straighten him out. He even gave him a new name of Paul, meaning —The little one‖ and appointed him to be the twelfth apostle. His task was the same as the other eleven men; they had to preach the Kingdom of Heaven, Yahshua being the King and they also had to heal the sick.

This —requested‖ fellow, Attorney Paul, after having spent three years in Heaven's seminary, where he received his education as a minister of the Gospel worked zealously day and night traveling all over to the countries where the scattered sheep of God were, preaching and healing, He also appointed

59

helpers, some evangelists, some preachers and elders and deacons etc. One such helper was Timothy, a real hardworking evangelist who suffered from stomach ulcers. Now when Paul had heard of this infirmity of Tim, he wrote him a letter in which he wrote 1 Timothy 5:2 Be no longer a drinker of water, but use a little wine for thy stomach's sake and thine often infirmities. Now what do you know! This was 2000 years ago. Over 80 times in the Old Testament wine is quoted as part of the important diet for man, as well as warnings against drowning yourself in the good stuff.

Like any prescription for medicine, it should be taken by measures: Psalms 104:15 And wine that maketh glad the heart of man, and oil to make his face to shine, and bread which strengtheneth man's heart. But keep to the instructions and do not be attempting to take an overdose.

Viva la vino!

Why not prevent rather than cure?

Remarkable! It was only yesterday that Dr. Marc Segal told on Fox about tests with red wine in Australia. Test results showed that men over 50 benefited greatly by drinking 4 ounces of red wine per day; they had an increase in bone strength and a good blood flow and pressure. Dr. Segal went on to say that a good example is the European nations like Italy enjoy a healthier life and far less heart problems.

—Bacon and Eggs, please‖

A cause of cancer. During my more than 80 years as a resident on this globe, I have read many publications on the research on the consumption of pork; so a few more won't harm you; after all, a few hours reading might just keep you above ground a decade or two longer and save you the agony of suffering with excruciating cancerous pain. Millions of such orders for breakfast are executed on a daily basis. So much so that the only place where a pig's life is not endangered is in Jerusalem; may be. It seems that the only tribe of Israel that complies with the Hygiene laws is Judah.

USA TODAY 2007, this article appeared:

—There is more evidence than ever that a person who weighs too much is more likely to develop cancer, a landmark report said Wednesday.
And forget eating bacon, sausage and ham. No amount is considered safe, according to the analysis from the American Institute for Cancer Research and the World Cancer Research Fund.

An international panel of experts reviewed more than 7,000 large-scale studies and spent five years developing the report.

Excess body fat increases the risk of cancer of the colon, kidney, pancreas, esophagus and uterus as well as postmenopausal breast cancer, the report says.‖

"This was a much larger impact than even the researchers expected," says Karen Collins, a cancer Institute nutrition adviser. "People forget body fat is not an inert glob that we are carrying around on the waistline and thighs. It's a metabolically active tissue that produces substances in the body that promote the development of cancer. "Michael Thune, head of epidemiological research for the American Cancer Society, says, "People are not paying nearly enough attention to the relationship between obesity and increased cancer risk." The report also found: Every 1.7 ounces of processed meat consumed a day increases the risk of colon rectal cancer by 21%.

"This is a wake-up call for people who eat hot dogs [Pork] or pepperoni [pork] pizza regularly," Collins says. "They need to be looking for other alternatives." All thus according to the USA Today report.

I remember having read an article in the South African Medical Journal when I was about fifteen years old, way back in 1942, that pork was a main cause of cancer. I showed the article to my pork eater family, but they just brushed it off. The article referred to tests that were done by some medical outfit in England that proved the cause of cancer by eating swine.

Elmer Jacobson, in his very informative book, entitled —God's Key To Health And Happiness‖ tells how he nearly lost his life due to cancer caused by pork. He gives an account of how he as a pastor had to suffer, simply because he did not honor the Creator's menu, but rather followed his own taste.

I am in my eighties and have refrained from eating pork since I was a small child. I just could never get around putting that stuff in my mouth. Perhaps it was because of the looks of the pig; or might just have been divinely so ordained. One evening, when I was about eight years old, my mother served soup that had some bacon in it. I ate one mouth full, and when I tasted the piece of bacon, I excused myself, ran for the bathroom and vomited; ever since I refrained from eating any form of pork Thanks be to God, for I have lived a very healthy life without hospitalization. I even still have all my teeth, appendix and tonsils. .

A pig and a hen were walking down the street and saw a sign on a door; the hen read it out loud —Fresh eggs and bacon for breakfast‖; the pig replied —Yup, for you it means a love offering but for me it means a blood sacrifice.‖

Filthy places are frequently referred to as —Pigsties‖. Having been raised on a self-sustaining farm where bacon and eggs or sausage and eggs was a regular breakfast diet, which meant me having only egg for this vital morning meal. Father raised amongst others, beef, mutton and poultry etc. The famous —Boerwors‖ sausage that was homemade, was mainly beef with some pork fat for better barbeque lubrication, and was well spiced up. What I am trying to tell you is that I know something about pigs. I even had to feed those swine. I have seen them in that filthy mud hole. At first, you distinguish nothing but a pile of black, slimy mud. The dirty mass moves! It always reminded me of a reptile, like a turtle or some uncouth monster, reveling in his stygian filth. A grunt! The mystery is solved. This describes the character of a pig/ hog/ swine. You avert your face and hasten by, sickened with disgust. Now my friend, does that make your mouth water for your savory ham, your pork chop, your tripe, your toothsome sausage or that crispy bacon in its native element? A dainty beast isn't he!

I borrow a clip from Mr. Josephson.

—Gaze over into that sty, our pork-eating friend. Have you done so before? And would you prefer to be excused? Quite likely; but we will show you a dozen things you did not observe before. See the contented brute quietly reposing in the augmented filth of his own odor! He seems to feel quite at home, doesn't he? Look a little sharper, and scrutinize his skin. Is it smooth and healthy? Not exactly so. So obscured is it by litter, and scurf, and mange, that you almost expect to see the rotten mass drop off as the grunting creature rubs it against any projecting corner which may furnish him a convenient scratching-place. As you glance around the pen, you observe that all such conveniences have been utilized until they are worn so smooth as to be almost inefficient.‖

In 1982 my family and I made a European tour by automobile; driving through the northern counties of Netherlands during the time of the Dutch farmers spreading hog manure on their flowerbeds, we were absolutely sickened by the odor hanging in the air. The pigsty is invariably placed quite a distance from the dwelling place precisely because of its perfume making process. Rouse the beast, and make him show his gait. See how he rolls along on a mountain of fat. If he were human, he would be advised to chew tobacco for his obesity, and would be expected to drop off any day of heart disease. And so he will do, unless the butcher forestalls nature by a few days. Indeed, not long ago a stout neighbor of his was quietly taking his breakfast from his trough, grunting his infinite satisfaction, when, without a moment's warning or a single premonitory symptom, his heart ceased to beat, and he instantly expired without finishing his meal, much to the disappointment of his owner, who was anticipating the pleasure of quietly executing him a few hours later, and serving him up to his pork-loving patrons. Suppose his death had been delayed a few hours, or rather, suppose the butcher had got the start of nature a little, as he generally contrives to do!

You can dress him up and put a golden ring in his snout and put him in a clean washed sty; it will simply change the outside of the swine yet not the inside. I have personally witnessed the wild boar where he has the open spaces at his disposal and what do you see, but a dirty swine rolling in the mud-hole then go around to see where there is some carcass for him to feast on; carrying out his function he was created to do. Pork-loving friend, take a nearer view of the animal that is destined to delight the palates of some of your friends, perhaps your own. Make him straighten out his fore legs. Take a close look and you see the open sore or issue, a few inches above his foot on the inner side? It is not a mere accidental abrasion? Find the same on the other leg; it is rather a wise and wonderful provision of nature. Grasp the leg high up and press downward. Now you see its utility, as a mass of corruption pours out. That opening is the outlet of a sewer. Yes, a scrofulous sewer; and hence the offensive matter which discharges from it. The pig enjoys the discharge by leaking the stuff.

Should you fill a syringe with mercury or some colored injecting fluid, and drive the contents into this same opening, you would be able to trace all through the body of the animal little pipes communicating with it.

What must be the condition of the body of an animal so foul as to require a regular system of drainage to convey away its teeming filth? Sometimes the accumulation of external filth closes the outlet. Then the ichorous stream ceases to flow, and the animal quickly sickens and dies unless the owner cleanses the parts, and so opens a new the feculent fountain, and allows the festering poison to escape.

What dainty morsels those same feet and legs make! What a delicate flavor they have, as every epicure asserts! Do you suppose the corruption with which they are saturated has any influence upon their taste and healthfulness?

Perhaps you are thoroughly disgusted now, and would like to leave the scene. Pause a moment. Now let us look at the inside of this wonderfully delicious beast!

You may rightfully ask me the question as to why did God create this filthy animal; the answer is simply for to be a scavenger.

Oink autopsy

Growing up on a farm during WW11 when soap was very scarce, I witnessed the making of soap from what they call —lard‖ derived from that slaughtered pig. At first the hog is held still, then the next thing is his sudden death caused by the hit of a hammer right between the eyes. Followed by boiling water over it to shave off the hog hair as strong as steel wires. The next repulsive act is the cutting open of the stomach area from where the guts are removed. Well, by then I as an eyewitness have long gone vanished to a secluded place, so as to escape me being culpable in that killing. Just under the foul and putrid skin we find a mass of fat from two to six inches in thickness, covering a large portion of the body. This stuff is then cooked on an open fire in a big black kaffer pot; that is a three-legged cast iron pot that holds about twenty five-gallons. It cooks all day during which time someone is stirring into the fat lye whilst coloring agent with some herbs added for odor. That soap was mainly used for laundry. Even if you put a nice red bow round his neck after having given him a bath, using the best shampoo, the inside of that pig remains unchanged. Do you imagine that the repulsiveness of this loathsome creature is only on the outside? That within everything is pure and wholesome? Vain delusion! Sickening, disgusting, as is the exterior, it is, in comparison with what it covers, a fair cloak, hiding a mass of disease and rottenness, which grows more superlatively filthy as we penetrate deeper and deeper beneath the skin.

Now what is this? Lard, says one; animal oil; an excellent thing for consumptives; a very necessary kind of food in cold weather. Lard, animal oil, very truly and, we will add a synonym for disease, scrofula, and torpid liver. Where did all that fat come from, or how happened it to be so heaped up around that poor hog? Surely it is not natural; for fat is only deposited in large quantities for the purpose of keeping the body warm in winter. This fat is much more than is necessary for such a purpose, and is much greater in amount than ever exists upon the animal in a state of nature. It is evidently the result of disease. So gross have been the habits of the animal, so great has been the foulness of its body, that its excretory organs--its liver, lungs, kidneys, skin, and intestines--have been entirely unable to carry away the impurities which the animal has been all its life accumulating. And even the extensive system of sewerage with its constant stream, which we have already described, was insufficient to the task of purging so vile a body of the debris, which abounded in every organ and saturated every tissue. Consequently this great flood of disease, which made its way through the veins and arteries into the tissues, and there accumulated as fat! Delectable morsel, a slice of fat pork, isn't it? Concentrated, consolidated filth!

Then the fatter the hog, the more diseased he is. Certainly. A few years ago, there were on exhibition at the great cattle show in England a couple of hogs which had been stuffed with oil cake until they were the greatest monsters of obesity ever exhibited. Of course, they took the first premium; and if a premium had been awarded to the animals, which were capable of producing the most disease, it is quite probable that they would have headed the list still.

Lard, then, obtained from the flesh of the hog by heating, is nothing more than extract of a diseased carcass! Who that knows its character would dare to defile him with this "broth of abominable things?"

Disgusting Developments: The hog.

Geoff Clark of the Brown Cancer Center — University of Louisville

—Now let us take a little deeper look, be prepared to find disease and corruption more abundant the deeper we go. Observe the glands, which lie about the neck. Instead of being of their ordinary size, and composed of ordinary gland structure, we find them surrounded by large masses of scrofulous tissue. Perhaps

67

tuberculosis degeneration had already taken place. If so, the soft, cheesy, infectious mass is ready to so broadcast the seeds of consumption and premature death. For, according to some excellent authorities, tuberculosis disease is capable of communication by means of tubercles. If the animal is of sufficient age, the further process of ulceration will have occurred.

Now take a deeper look still, and examine the lungs of this much-prized animal. If he is more than a few months old, you will be likely to find large numbers of tubercles. If he is much more than a year old, you will be more likely than not to find a portion of the lung completely consolidated. Yet all of this filthy, diseased mass is cooked as a delicious morsel, and served up to satisfy fastidious tastes. If the animal had escaped the butcher's knife a few years, he would have died of tuberculosis consumption.

But what kind of a liver would you expect such an animal to have? Is not excessive fatness one of the surest evidences of a diseased and inactive liver? Infallible! Then a fat hog must have a dreadfully diseased bile manufactory. Make a cut into its substance. In seventy-five cases out of a hundred you will find it filled with abscesses. In a larger percentage still will be found the same diseased products, which seem to infest every organ, every tissue, and every structure of the animal. Yet these same rotten, diseased, scrofulous livers are eaten and relished by thousands of people who cannot express their contempt for the Frenchman who eats a horse or the China man who dines upon fricasseed puppy.

Now just glance at the remaining contents of the abdomen. In every part you notice evidences, unmistakable, of scrofula, fatty degeneration, and tuberculosis masses.

Where Scrofula Comes From. The word —scrofula‖ is derived from the Latin scrofu, which means a sow. The ancient Romans evidently believed that scrofula originated with the hog, and hence they attached the name of the beast to the disease. Saying that a man has scrofula, then, is equivalent to saying that he has the hog disease. After we have seen that the hog is the very embodiment of scrofulous disease, can anyone doubt the accuracy of the conclusion of the Romans?

Origin of the Tapeworm

We shall attempt to trace the history of this horrid parasite only so far as concerns its introduction into the human system.

With this end in view, let us glance again at the diseased liver. It will be no uncommon thing if we discover numberless little sacs, or cysts, about the size of a hemp seed. These do not present a very formidable appearance, certainly, but, as soon as they are taken into the human stomach, the gastric juice dissolves off the membranous sac, and liberates a minute animal, which had been lurking there for months, perhaps, awaiting this very opportunity. This creature, although very small, is furnished with a head and four suckers, which attach themselves firmly to the wall of the intestine, and the parasite begins to grow. In a short time an addition to its body is produced posteriorly, attached like a joint. Soon a duplicate of this appears, and then another, and another, until the body attains a length of several yards. Not infrequently tapeworms measuring thirty to one hundred feet in length are found in the intestines of human beings.

Under some circumstances the eggs of the tapeworm find entrance into the body, when the disease is developed in another form. The embryonic worms consist of a pair of hooklets so shaped that a twisting motion will cause them to penetrate the tissues after the fashion of a corkscrew. Countless numbers of these may be taken into the system, since a single tapeworm has been found to produce more than two million eggs. By the boring motion referred to, which seems to be spontaneous in the young worm, the parasites penetrate into every part of the body. Penetrating the walls of the blood vessels, they are swept along in the life-current, thus finding their way even to the most delicate structures of the human system. They have been found in all the organs of the body, even the brain and the delicate organs of vision not escaping the depredations of this destructive parasite.

When this lively migrating germ gets fully settled in the tissues, it becomes enveloped in a little cell, and remains quiet until taken into the stomach of some other animal, when it is liberated, and speedily develops into a full-grown tapeworm, as already described. But although quiet, the imprisoned parasite is by no means harmless. The cysts formed often attain such a size as to endanger life. When developed in the eye, they occasion blindness; in the lungs or other organs, they interfere with the proper functions of the organs; in the liver, which is the frequent rendezvous of these destructive creatures, a most serious and fatal disease known as hydatid is occasioned by the extraordinary development of the cysts, which are originally not larger than a pea, but by excessive growth assume enormous proportions. The same disease may occur in any other part of the body in which the germs undergo development.

The germs of these dreadful animals are found not only in the liver, but in other organs as well. Pork containing them is said to be "measly." Sometimes the condition is discovered; but that such is not always the case is evidenced by the fact that tapeworm is every year becoming more frequent. It has long been common in Germany. In Iceland it has become extremely common. In Abyssinia the occurrence of the worm has become so frequent, owing to the bad dietetic habits of the people, that it has been said that every Abyssinian has a tapeworm. In this country the parasite is most common among butchers and cooks.

Some time since, we received from a friend in the South a specimen of pork which was so densely peopled with the germs of this dreadful parasite that every cubic inch of flesh contained more than a score of them. The writer has in his microscope cabinet specimens of the embryonic worms taken from hydatid tumors of the liver of a patient who died of the disease in Bellevue Hospital, New York.

The poor victim who is forced to entertain this unwelcome guest suffers untold agonies, and finally dies, if he cannot succeed in dislodging the parasite.

The Terrible Trichina

Now, my friend, assist your eyesight by a good microscope, and you will be convinced that you have only just caught a glimpse of the enormous filthiness, the inherent badness, and the intrinsic ugliness of this loathsome animal. Take a thin slice of lean flesh; place it upon the stage of your microscope, adjust the eyepiece, and look. You will see displayed before your eyes hundreds of voracious little animals, each coiled up in its little cell, waiting for an opportunity to escape from its prison walls and begin its destined work of devastation.

A Prominent man in Louisville has made extensive researches upon the subject, and asserts that in at least one hog out of every ten these creatures may be found. A committee appointed by the Chicago Academy of Medicine to investigate this subject reported that they found in their examinations at the various packinghouses in the city, one hog in fifty infested with trichina. Other investigations have shown a still greater frequency of the disease.

Some years ago I obtained a small portion of the flesh of a person who had died from trichina poisoning. Upon subjecting it to a careful microscopic examination with a good instrument, [Thanks again to Leeuwenhoek] I discovered multitudes of little worms. Each individual presented the appearance shown in the accompanying accurate engraving. The animal is there seen enclosed in a little cyst, or sac, which is dissolved by the gastric juice when taken into the stomach. The parasite, being thus set at liberty, immediately penetrates the thin muscular walls of the stomach, and gradually works its way through the whole muscular system. It possesses the power of propagating its species with wonderful rapidity; and a person once infected is almost certain to die a lingering death of excruciating agony.

In Helmstadt, Prussia, one hundred and three persons were poisoned in this way, and twenty of them died within a month.

It is doubtless not known how many deaths are really due to this cause; for many persons die of strange, unknown diseases, which baffle the doctors? Still both as to cure and diagnosis. Trichinosis very much resembles various other diseases in some of its stages, and is likely to be attributed to other than its true cause. It is

Thought, by prominent medical men, that hundreds of people die of the disease without suspecting its true nature.

Published: Jun. 9, 2010

Source: Laurie Rund, Published: Jun. 9, 2010

University of Illinois researchers believe the pig may hold answers for scientists studying breast cancer, a disease that kills 500,000 women worldwide each year.

While extraordinary advances in the understanding of cancer's molecular basis have occurred in the past 10 years, current models for drug testing are not keeping pace.

"The failure of current animal models to predict the human response is a critical bottleneck and is likely to become the limiting factor in the development of effective new cancer therapies," said Laurie Rund, U of I research assistant professor in animal sciences. "In order to take advantage of the advances in novel therapeutic design, we need to find a more physiological and predictive animal model for cancer."

Rund and U of I colleague Lawrence Schook, in collaboration with Jason Chesney and principal investigator Geoff Clark of the Brown Cancer Center — University of Louisville, have been awarded a National Institutes of Health EUREKA (Exceptional, Unconventional Research Enabling Knowledge Acceleration) grant to develop a transgenic swine model for cancer.

Under the four-year project entitled, "Oncopigs as a Better Model for Human Cancer," collaborators will use state-of-the-art technology to generate transgenic pigs that can be induced to lose the expression of three major tumor suppressors simultaneously in the breast.

"These genetic defects are often found in breast cancer, particularly in Triple Negative breast cancer," Rund said. "Triple Negative breast cancer is especially aggressive and difficult to treat. It has a high morbidity rate and affects African American women at almost three times the rate of the general population."

Rund and her teammates have already discovered that it takes five to six genetic defects to convert a normal pig cell into a tumor cell — just like humans. However, mouse cells, which have been used in many previous studies, can be transformed into tumor cells by as little as two genetic defects.

72

In addition, pigs are similar to humans because they can live for decades and have a very low rate of spontaneous cancer. This is in contrast to rodent-based cancer models, where life span is limited to a few years and the spontaneous development of cancer is high.

Rund said this study could allow their team to validate the pig as a superior model to study human cancer.

"If this works, we can study more types of cancer using the pig model," Rund said. "It's the first transgenic pig model for breast cancer that I know of, although pigs have been used extensively in biomedical research for years."

Investigators testing novel, unconventional hypotheses or major methodological or technical challenges are sought after to receive NIH Eureka grants.

"Only 30 EUREKA grants are awarded each year," said Lawrence Schook, Gutgsell professor of animal sciences and director of the Division of Biomedical Sciences. "We are honored to receive this award as it targets exceptionally innovative research that will have a substantial impact on the scientific community."

It is a well known fact that scavengers, that is to say, animals, such as the hog, the elephant etc; that do not chew the cud, have an incomplete digestive system which explains why their bodies absorb, instead of discharging the sinister parasites. They are minute spiral worms which scientists call —trichinella spiralis.‖ One scientist wrote, —A single serving of infected pork, yes even a single mouthful can kill or cripple or condemn a victim to a lifetime of aches and pains.‖ For this unique disease, trichinoses, there is no sure cure. According to Dr. Laird Goldberg.

Let me just say that even if the pig should wear a pink bow round his neck and a golden ring in his snout, it is the filthiest thing about.

Bon appetite!

Maker's Handbook and the oink, oink

The omniscient Creator of this complicated earth system with its cosmos arranged a complete, self-sustaining self-cleansing operation. The result of life inevitably produces waste; for example, take the cow that consumes vast amount of fodder daily will drop daily heaps of manure that need cleaning; for this purpose He created the manure beetles.   Having been raised on an African farm, I always noticed that when walking in the veld you never see any skeletons lying about, despite the fact that the tigers had only recently killed some baboons. So, you wonder what happened to the many bones. Ah! Let me tell you; the scavengers did their work. First, when the tiger or lion had finished its meal, the vultures had picked the bones clean. Now there were still left the intestines, the hide and the bones. So there came along the hyenas and the wolves and they ate the bones. The hide was often left to the hog that would leave it to rot and then feat on it. The pig thrives on rotten stuff. Oh, then comes along you and eat the pig. How ghastly!!

What I am trying to convey to my readers is the fact that Almighty God created a wonderful balance in nature. Man is His pride creature and He speaks to man telling him what to eat and what not to eat. Even in His instructions to father Noah He makes provision for food during and after the flood or then deluge. Noah had to accommodate in that floating hotel seven pairs of the —Clean animals‖ whereas only one pair of the rest of the animal kingdom. Genesis 7:1 And the Lord said unto Noah, Come thou and all thy house into the ark; for thee have I seen righteous before me in this generation. 2. Of every clean beast thou shalt take to thee by sevens, the male and his female: and of beasts that are not clean by two, the male and his female. So, it proves that the command to Moses was not new at all.

I have reason to believe that father Noah and family liked their chicken, thank Goodness, because just think what Colonel Sanders would have done without the feathered friends: God still speaking to our ancestor saying in verse 3: Of fowls also of the air by sevens, the male and the female; to keep seed alive upon the face of all the earth.

Hello! Are you going to finish that bacon? I anticipate your next question, which is, —But where does God say that the swine is unclean? Now I wonder just how many quotes you will need to be convinced. Let's see:

Now this is at least 800 years after the flood and before the only one tribe of Israel, namely Judah was nicknamed —Jew. In all fairness to the Tribe of Benjamin, they were also reckoned to be Judeans or Juds or Jews. Now God is addressing the ancestors of the Church, that is to say the Elect or ecclesia. The clean animals for human consumption: Leviticus 11:1 And the Lord spake unto Moses and to Aaron, saying unto them, 1. And the Lord spake unto Moses and to Aaron, saying unto them, 2. Speak unto the children of Israel, saying, These are the beasts which ye shall eat among all the beasts that are on the earth. 3. Whatsoever parteth the hoof, and is clovenfooted, and cheweth the cud, among the beasts, that shall ye eat.   The unclean animals: 4. Nevertheless these shall ye not eat of them that chew the cud, or of them that divide the hoof: as the camel, because he cheweth the cud, but divideth not the hoof; he is unclean unto you. 5. And the coney, because he cheweth the cud, but divideth not the hoof; he is unclean unto you. 6. And the hare, because he cheweth the cud, but divideth not the hoof; he is unclean unto you. 7 And the swine, though he divide the hoof, and be clovenfooted, yet he cheweth not the cud; he is unclean to you. 8 Of their flesh shall ye not eat, and their carcase shall ye not touch; they are unclean to yo!.

Oh my friend, so many people get so sick just because they ignore Yahweh's laws and find all clever excuses for doing so. I have witnessed more than one minister of the Lord feasting on prohibited food such as ham, sausage and catfish. Just as God was concerned for the welfare of Noah et al, He still is concerned for our safety today. He gives us a Menu to follow. As is detailed in the book of Leviticus chapter seven. Do yourself a favor and study it carefully, memorizing it; do it my friend, it is for your own good.

How many times have I heard a sick person saying —If it is God's will He will heal me‖ but in the same time he or she defies God's Laws. He is rightly the Elohim that heals us. People are inclined to pick and choose the portion of Scripture that suits them and apply that to their prayers. Believe me dear reader, I do not mean to be nasty; I am just trying to direct God's beloved creatures to the truth as the truth will set us free. Yes even from diseases such as cancer If: Exodus 15:26 And said, <u>If</u> thou wilt diligently hearken to the voice of the Lord thy God, and wilt <u>do that which is right</u> in his sight, and wilt <u>give ear to his commandments, and keep all his statutes, I will put none of these diseases upon thee</u>, which I have brought upon the Egyptians: <u>for I AM the Lord that healeth thee.</u> It is this last phrase that believers pick for favorite and leave out the rest with the —IF‖.

Now if you still want to be obstreperous and stubborn like a mule, and say as so many do —Oh that what you quote is from the Old Testament, and does not apply to us for today.— My answer will be outright —OK, go ahead and kill and steal and lie and just break all the Ten Commandments for they are all out of the Old Testament. No, my friend, He that said you shall not commit adultery also said you must not eat swine etc. As we know from military terms, a command is stronger than a law. The Big Ten are mere headings for all that follow.

The next thing you will refer to is in the New Testament where Peter saw the great sheet descending from Heaven and saw all the four legged animals in that sheet and a voice said —go ahead Peter kill and eat.‖ So you are also one of those that twist and turn like a blacksmith twists iron. Sorry buddy, that sheet was not a menu but an indication to Peter that he had to go to the other tribes [Gentiles] that were not recognized by the southern two tribes for this new Messianic Faith. The variety of clean and unclean animals meant the variety of nations, which the northern ten tribes, scattered among the nations, became. The first one of the Lost Sheep he met was Cornelius, a Roman captain, who feared Yahweh but had not heard of Yahshua the Messiah. Oh, and

76

another point to be considered is the fact that Scripture says all four legged animals, that tells me that if that were a menu, there would have been under the all some sheep etc. Approximately seven years after Pentecost this vision came to Peter whilst he was meditating on the roof, sending him to the house of Cornelius, the Gentile. But, though he obeyed God, until this time they had preached the Word exclusively but unto the Jews, that is to say Judah and Benjamin. The reason being that the northern Ten Tribes were by this time of the apostles out of sight and had been out of mind for over seven hundred years, and were not being reckoned as part of Israel, in fact the northern ten tribes were despised by the Judeans even before their dispersement. What Peter did not realize was that Yahweh had made an everlasting covenant with all twelve tribes of Jacob. Later on in Peter's epistle he directs his writings to all twelve 1 Peter 1:1

Peter, an apostle of Jesus Christ, to the elect who are sojourners of the Dispersion in Pontus, Galatia, Cappadocia, Asia, and Bithynia,

The Bible witnesses the same about the other apostles see James 1:1 James, a servant of God and of the Lord Jesus Christ, to the twelve tribes which are scattered abroad, greeting.

Honest Questions must be asked and searched from Scripture about all these matters; so let us without prejudice open our minds and search diligently for the truth. First, let us remember this Heavenly vision with all kind of unclean beasts came down from Heaven. The Lord did not show him only unclean animals such as pigs. It is essential that we bear in mind that the sheet was caught up again into heaven. Now, did the words, "Rise, Peter, kill and eat," mean that God was repealing the dietary laws? Is God reversing Himself on physical hygiene and sanitation in His requirement that a clean people have clean food? Did Messiah's work on the cross perform a biological miracle in these filthy scavenger animals that made their flesh harmless to eat and fit for human consumption? Did the dispensation of grace and the coming of the gospel so alter the gastric processes and digestive apparatus of man that all unclean meats will now build healthy bodies instead of producing disease and result in death as they did before?

Peter's Conclusion

According to verse 17, Peter himself was a little mystified as to what the meaning of this vision was as we read in verse I7; —Peter doubted in himself what this vision which he had seen should mean." There is not a shadow of inkling, as the context clearly proves, that Peter believed this vision had anything to do with a change in the dietary law. The unclean beasts, fowls and creeping things were symbols of those scattered tribes of long time ago. The animals in discussion were representative of nations, similar to the symbols of today where USA has an eagle as an emblem, Britain has a Lion as their emblem, Russia has a Bear for their emblem, China has a snake representing them, and South Africa has a Springbok, the only clean animal of the mentioned. And so on and so forth. At this point in time, the Ten as well as many of the two Tribes were to be found all over the world, amongst the Nations of the world. We read in Deuteronomy 30 1. And it shall come to pass, when all these things are come upon thee, the blessing and the curse, which I have set before thee, and thou shalt call them to mind among all the nations, whither the Lord thy God hath driven thee, 2. And shalt return unto the Lord thy God, and shalt obey his voice according to all that I command thee this day, thou and thy children, with all thine heart, and with all thy soul; 3. That then the Lord thy God will turn thy captivity, and have compassion upon thee, and will return and gather thee from all the nations, whither the Lord thy God hath scattered thee. 4. If any of thine be driven out unto the outmost parts of heaven, from thence will the Lord thy God gather thee, and from thence will he fetch thee:
Yahweh had told Father Abraham that his seed would become many nations; well, they did; just consider the salami of nations we have in the good old US of A. Then, there is the New

Covenant promise in Jeremiah 31: 31.   Behold, the days come, saith the Lord, that I will make a new covenant with the house of Israel, and with the house of Judah: 32.   Not according to the covenant that I made with their fathers in the day that I took them by the hand to bring them out of the land of Egypt; which my covenant they break, although I was an husband unto them, saith the Lord: 33.   But this shall be the covenant that I will make with the house of Israel; After those days, saith the Lord, I will put my law in their inward parts, and write it in their hearts; and will be their God, and they shall be my people.34.   And they shall teach no more every man his neighbor, and every man his brother, saying, Know the Lord: for they shall all know me, from the least of them unto the greatest of them, saith the Lord: for I will forgive their iniquity, and I will remember their sin no more. Messiah kept His promise of a New Covenant and instituted it Himself on occasion of the Last Supper Luke 22:20 And the cup in like manner after supper, saying, This cup is the new covenant in my blood, even that which is poured out for many.

Now dear reader, if this does not convince you that Peter's vision was not a menu a la carte pertaining to hogs and monkeys, then nothing will. I have more news for the pork lovers, and that is that my Savior kept the law and even fulfilled it to the last dot. Now you can go ahead and commit suicide if you like. You have been warned of that lingering imminent danger. Why must man always tease God?

1 Samuel 15:23 for rebellion [Obstinate] is as the sin of witchcraft, and stubbornness is as idolatry and teraphim. Because thou hast rejected the word of Yahweh, he hath also rejected thee from being king.

. Scavengers were never created for human consumption. The God-given law to Moses condemns this meat, manufactured out of the filthiest and most abominable matter, as unclean. In its very nature it is poisonous, diseased and deadly. The flesh of the swine is said by many authorities to be the prime cause of much of our American ill health, causing blood diseases, weakness of the stomach, liver troubles, eczema, consumption, tumors, cancer, etc. The Law of Yahweh He instructed the Hebrew nations to consider all other Goyim, pagan nations unclean.

Messiah came to save His people from their sin, ergo, cleanse them by the washing in His Blood. He came to fulfill His promise as described in the New Covenant. 2 Thessalonians 3: and that we may be delivered from bad and evil men, for faith is not the portion of all. We must bear in mind that the Jews have disinherited the Northern Ten Tribes long ago, 720 B.C. and reckoned them as heathen, ergo, unclean. Oh! The omniscient God; He knows exactly where His sheep are and He will carry out His promises in the Everlasting Covenant to the minutest details.

We witnessed the fact that Peter's vision was not a menu a la carte but a show of all Israel scattered amongst the unclean nations. After seven hundred years of being scattered amongst the nations of the world, they were completely assimilated and even spoke in those tongues; and apart from the fact the Lord was telling him not to hesitate to "arise and eat" with these unclean Gentiles, for the sake of sharing the world-inclusive Messianic message with them.

Peter's own testimony regarding the vision was, "God hath showed me that I should not call any MAN [not animal] common or unclean." Cornelius, an Italian, was of one of the nations, which the Jews had considered unclean. Later, when the church officials at Jerusalem called Peter on the carpet, they contended with him and accused him of going "into men un-circumcised, and did eat with them." Uncircumcision was a mark of uncleanness. If a man [Jewish or proselyte] was not circumcised, he was cut off from God's covenant. In the 11th chapter of Acts, Peter rehearsed the matter to the apostles, who were shocked that he would associate with one of an unclean nation. He testified that, as he spoke the Word of God, the Spirit of God from heaven fell on these "unclean," and that they experienced the same wonderful cleansing that they themselves had received. Peter commanding them to be baptized in the Name of Yahshua the Messiah symbolized this cleansing. Messiah had told His apostles that His SHEEP know His Voice; that is to say when we preach the Word, those that come are fit for acceptance into the Church, since only the Holy Spirit can make you believe. Again may I refer you to the New Covenant that says —I will put My Spirit in them and…‖

 It is worthy, also, to consider that Cornelius was a —God Fearer', evidently an Israelite descendant of the Northern Tribes.   I say this because Scripture tells us that he was a man of prayer. It is clear that this man Cornelius was one of the so called lost Sheep of Israel of whom Yahshua spoke when He said [Darby's Bible] Matthew 10:5 These twelve Jesus sent out when he had charged them, saying, Go not off into the way of the nations, and into a city of Samaritans enter ye not; 6. But go rather to the lost sheep of the house of Israel.

The above mentioned has a lot to do with our health, in that we learn about the concern the Almighty Creator has for His elected people.   So, whether you consider yourself one of the elect or not, you can at least learn what is good for your health and what is not.

From the love of the Savior's heart He calls His elect sheep, after that very kind little animal that would always follow the shepherd. I sometimes wonder whether we really deserve such a kind name, instead of a more appropriate name of —His Pigs‖ after that filthy animal that eat anything.

But wait! There is more to come.

Fish

"The good, the bad and the ugly." I mean real ugly. Some anyway.

Is it not weird that we as human beings are by nature inclined to do just the opposite from what is right? As is stated in the Heidelberg Catechism. —We are by nature inclined to hate God and neighbor.‖ When are we going, if ever, to learn to prefer the good to the bad? Have you ever watched a crab walking? He does not walk straight but always sideways. I recall in my boyhood how I disliked, with angst, those crabs when fishing and how they took the bait and ran with it and I, with great expectation reeled in; only to be disappointed with either nothing on the hook or one of them ghastly creatures waving his legs and popping his little eyes with his pinchers wide open and ready to clip your finger. But, sometimes I was too quick for that ugly crab; when I pull up he was to slow to let go and he landed on solid ground where he met his fate. I detest seeing them arabesque creatures on diner's plates in restaurants. What I actually mean to say is that the way we walk will be the way that our children walk. As the saying goes, —Like father, like son and like mother, like daughter.‖

Another nasty little tasty creature that can cause your demise is the shrimp. It was many years ago that, one day I read in the Natal Mercury about people that had died suddenly from arsenic poisoning after having eaten shrimps. I then learned that those little scavengers, closely related to crabs, lobsters and crayfish all pose a similar danger. Then you just wonder why would people develop a taste for things that must be dressed up for taste in preference of real delicious fish that is not only wholesome but also naturally very tasty.

Glancing the web, I stumbled on an article that read: In Taiwan, a woman suddenly died unexpectedly with signs of bleeding from her ears, nose, mouth & eyes. After a preliminary autopsy, it was diagnosed death due to arsenic poisoning. Where did the arsenic come from? The police launched an in-depth and extensive investigation. A medical school professor was invited to come to solve the case. The professor carefully looked at the contents from the deceased's stomach, in less than half an hour, the mystery was solved. The professor said: 'the deceased did not commit suicide and neither was she murdered, she died of accidental death due to ignorance!' Everyone was puzzled, why accidental death? The professor said: 'The arsenic is produced in the stomach of the deceased.' The deceased used to take 'Vitamin C' everyday, which in itself is not a problem. The problem was that she ate a large portion of shrimp/prawn during dinner. Eating shrimp/prawn is not the problem that's why nothing happened to her family even though they took the same shrimp/prawn. However at the same time the deceased also took 'vitamin C', that is where the problem is!

Researchers at the University of Chicago in the United States, found through experiments, food such as soft-shell shrimp/prawn contains a much higher concentration of - five potassium arsenic compounds. Such fresh food by itself has no toxic effects on the human body! However, in taking 'vitamin C', due to the chemical reaction, the original non-toxic - five potassium arsenic (As anhydride, also known as arsenic oxide, the chemical formula for As_2O_5) changed to a three potassium toxic arsenic (ADB arsenic anhydride), also known as arsenic trioxide, a chemical formula (As_2O_3), which is commonly known as arsenic to the public! Arsenic poisoning have magma role and can cause paralysis to the small blood vessels, inhibits the activity of the liver and fat necrosis change Hepatic Lobules Center, heart, liver, kidney, intestine congestion, epithelial cell necrosis, telangiectasia. Therefore, a person who dies of arsenic poisoning will show signs of bleeding from the ears, nose, mouth & eyes. Therefore; as a precautionary measure, DO NOT; not eat shrimp/prawn when taking 'vitamin C'. In itself it is rather silly and stupid, because we take vitamin C all day from our food and drinks.

At 31,500 species, fish exhibit greater species diversity than any other class of vertebrates. Out of such gigantic variety there are however, like in the animal kingdom, some species that are there for another purpose than to be available for the table. Having such a wide choice for the eater it is hard to understand why some people still are so naive as to pay exorbitant fees for dietetic advice, given by imperfect dietitians who are limited in knowledge?

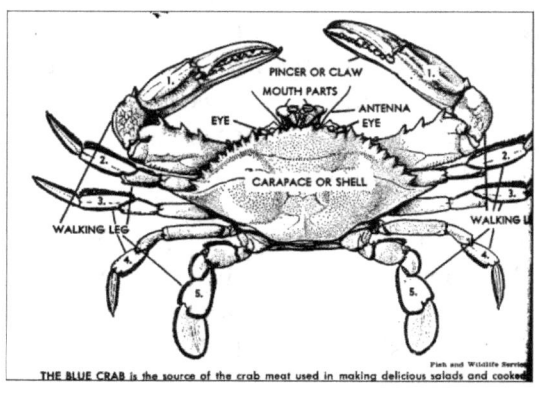

THE BLUE CRAB is the source of the crab meat used in making delicious salads and cooked

I prefer to consult the Maker of every living creature to get the best information as to what is safe for my body, such as any aquatic vertebrate animal that is covered with scales and equipped with two sets of paired fins. And so we read from the Maker's Handbook as penned by His servant Moses, circa four thousand years ago.

I have seen catfish shops where people line up for a seat to gulp up those scale less creatures. Don't they know? Or don't they care what God says about eating those aquatic scavengers. I believe that once you hear what He says that one should quit eating the stuff that can harm the temple of God. Food poisoning occurs when you eat food contaminated with bacteria or other toxins. Symptoms include diarrhea, vomiting, and stomach cramps, and generally start 4 - 36 hours after eating contaminated food. While bacteria often cause food poisoning, it can also result from eating poisonous plants (some mushrooms, for instance) and animals (puffer fish). Every year, more than 75 million people get sick from food poisoning, especially during summer when food may not be kept cold enough to prevent bacteria from growing.

It is also essential for our own welfare to observe the dietary law regarding the clean fish identified by fins and scales. Among these we have a large variety of such fish as the bass, pike, sunfish, perch, salmon, tuna, etc. Leviticus 11:9 these may ye eat of all that are in the waters: whatsoever hath fins and scales in the waters, in the seas, and in the rivers, that may ye eat. 10. And all that have not fins and scales in the seas, and in the rivers, of all that move in the waters, and of any living thing which is in the waters, they shall be an abomination unto you:

11. They shall be even an abomination unto you; ye shall not eat of their flesh, but ye shall have their carcasses in abomination. Whatsoever hath no fins nor scales in the waters, that shall be an abomination unto you.

As a fervent scholar of Scripture, I find nowhere any other recommendation in the Laws of God than what is recommended or actually commanded us by Him, all for our own good.

Our Role model is our beloved King Yahshua the Messiah; He always set the example for us. Nowhere do you find Him eating pork or lobsters or anything alike. On the contrary, He multiplied the couple of tilapia freshwater fishes enough to feed an entire congregation. And they that had eaten were about five thousand men, beside women and children.

Kentucky Fried Chicken is as American as is a John Wayne movie. The old colonel surely knew the Laws of God Yahweh, otherwise he probably would have cooked up —Kentucky barbequed pork ribs.‖

I remember as a young farm boy, father told me to shoot with my air gun only doves for us boys to cook on the open fire there in the bush; for he said that other birds are unclean and some even poisonous.

The unclean fowls which are prohibited for human consumption, are named in the dietary law, as given in Leviticus chapter ii. And these ye shall have in abomination among the birds; they shall not be eaten, they are an abomination: the eagle, and the gier-eagle, and the ospray. {Ostrich] 14. And the vulture, and the kite after his kind;

15. Every raven after his kind;

16. And the owl, and the night hawk, and the cuckow, and the hawk after his kind,

17. And the little owl, and the cormorant, and the great owl,

18. And the swan, and the pelican, and the gier eagle,

19. And the stork, the heron after her kind, and the lapwing, and the bat.

20. All fowls that creep, going upon all four, shall be an abomination unto you.

Some fowl such as geese, ducks, chickens and turkeys are clean by virtue of the gizzard that separates and cleanses all matter before it becomes flesh. Now here is that which was created for our consumption as was told by the Almighty Creator to Moses to tell us: YAHWEH speaks: Leviticus 11:21 Yet these may ye eat of all winged creeping things that go upon all fours, which have legs above their feet, wherewith to leap upon the earth.

Eating Fat

Reta, my wife and I went shopping in Amsterdam one evening when there were many people lingering on the side-walks; she made an observation —The Hollanders all seem to be slim and well dressed, but when you hear American English spoken, invariably the speaker is fat and sloppy.‖ I had to concur.

My brother, two years my junior, is a lover of fat mutton, fat beef of the finest quality. I mean the meat, whether it is muttonchops or any other meat dish must be loaded with a thick layer of fat. My late father and late brother, just older than I, both died of coronary thrombosis and they were also lovers of fat.

[Like all of us, they loved good eating. Father died at the age of 78 and brother died at the age of 64; they both died of coronary thrombosis.] My younger brother received six bypasses of the arteries, all on same day, at the age of 76. When he recovered from that ordeal, the hospital menu was presented to him, looking at it, he said, —Bring me steak with thick fat or nothing.‖ Well now, let me add this about my little brother, he burns that fatty meat by walking at a fast pace, four miles every day of the week, and believe me, it is not window shopping. He makes his own beef sausage, which he stuffs with pork fat. He loves ham and bacon. So there you have it. You be the judge.

How come we seem to have a family history of heart disease? Well it is not uncommon. In fact when you fill out that form at your doc's office you see that the question about a family history of heart disease is asked. Medical science has come a long way by research on this problem. They have established for a fact that animal fat is a cause of the accumulation of plaque in the arteries. And I suppose since we all eat the same food dished up on the same table, we all eat the same amount of fat. As the saying goes, —Like father like son.‖ Some people are wise and others just plain otherwise, and that goes for me. As I said before, I was never a neither fat nor pork eater.

My little brother was raised with animals and so was I, with a difference of him being a natural farmer and I being an engineer. When a beef or sheep was killed for the pot, I could never stand the sight of blood; consequently I made myself scarce from the abattoir. There was never a shortage of meat in our home; my parents' farm produced virtually everything bar things like coffee, tea and sugar. We had lots of all kinds of fruit and vegetables. Daddy, also, had a cattle ranch in the lowveld area where he moved the cattle for winter where pastures were favorable with lots of fodder. At that lowveld farm was a great variety of game, antelope like Kudu and wildebeest were plentiful. My father used to be an enthusiastic hunter made sure that we always had lots of —Biltong‖, known in America as jerky. I was and still am very fond of real South African jerky, preferably made from Kudu or springbok. Venison is healthy meat with a very low fat content. I, also, love fish and poultry. Now I do not wish to imply that I am immune to heart attack. But I can state that I have been blessed with a life without any serious illness, at least for my first eighty-two years. It is now in my eighty third year that I needed a stent and a pacemaker. I am still walking around with all my teeth, tonsils and appendix. The pace maker became necessary as a result of a slow heartbeat. I love to walk fast every day and then I get very tired because of a lack of oxygen being the result of the heart pulse's lagging behind the required pace. We are very fortunate here in North East Tennessee to have one of the top rated heart hospitals in the country. It rates within the top ten.

Usually, the blockage develops slowly and steadily over time. Plaque, made from cholesterol and other cells, thickens within the coronary artery walls. If the blood cannot flow through this blockage, you will experience a heart attack. Sometimes, the plaque in the arteries will tear and stick to blood platelets, forming a clot. A heart attack will occur if the clot prevents the blood from flowing.

You might experience a heart attack during moments of overwhelming stress or when you are physically exerting yourself while exercising. An illness such as pneumonia can also cause a heart attack. Many people experience heart attacks in the morning, suggesting that one possible cause involves the rhythm of platelets. My late father died of a heart attack whilst suffering an attack of pneumonia.

Both men and women can develop a heart attack. While men tend to experience more obvious symptoms, women will suffer from silent heart attacks without any symptoms at all. Most men become at risk in their mid-40s, and most women become at risk in their mid-50s. A family history of heart attacks and coronary artery disease can provide some indication of whether you are at risk. Individuals with a mother, father, brother, or sister who have suffered heart attacks are at risk.

Diabetes, obesity, high cholesterol, and high blood pressure are conditions that can trigger a heart attack. As a result, it is important that patients monitor these conditions and start treatment promptly, if necessary. I am not a medical doctor, but do get my information from those wonderful learnt fellows.

Diet and lifestyle can also put you at risk for a heart attack. Animal fat is probably the biggest culprit. Tobacco smokers and alcohol drinkers can put themselves at risk for a heart attack. People who do not exercise and live a sedentary lifestyle may develop a heart attack if they are considered overweight. All according to medical science. More than one school of learning, like the University of California issued bulletins on this subject, which corroborates the dietary law that God gave to Moses over fourteen hundred years before Christ. The bulletin by California University describes how the fatty protein molecules travel in the blood stream, and are deposited on the inner wall of the coronary artery. The proteins and fats are burned off, and the cholesterol is left behind. As it piles up, it narrows and irritates the artery, encouraging more formation of such deposits. It isn't long before the blood does not have sufficient room to flow freely through the veins and capillaries, and therefore, a high blood pressure condition is created which often results in a heart attack.

Tapping the brains of the experts:

Poly-unsaturated fat (unsaturated fat): There are two types of poly-unsaturated fat, omega-6 and omega-3 fats. Since most

Americans get plenty of omega-6 fats in their diet from vegetable oils, Dr. Schmitt says her primary concern is omega-3 fats. Good sources of omega-3 fats are fish (salmon and tuna), flaxseed, and walnuts.

Tip: Snack on a handful of walnuts, or add a tablespoon of ground flaxseed to your morning oatmeal or cereal. You can add ground flaxseed when you are baking cookies or muffins for an omega boost.

Saturated fat: Red meat, fatty meats like salami, dairy products such as cream and butter, and thicker vegetable oils like coconut, palm, and kernel oil are sources of saturated fats.

Tip: Enjoy a steak now and then, but try to limit saturated fats to 10 percent of your diet, at the most.

Trans fat: Made by adding hydrogen to vegetable oil, a process designed to extend the shelf life of packaged goods, trans fat is found in a wide range of packaged and processed foods, including bakery items, cookies, and crackers.

Tip: Current Food and Drug Administration guidelines allow manufacturers to say that their product is "trans fat free" if it contains less than 0.5 grams of trans fat per serving. Check the labels of processed food for "hydrogenated" or "partially hydrogenated" oils in the ingredients. These words signal that product may have up to 0.5 grams per serving. Eat a few servings, and this starts to add up. The above research and discoveries over the past century or more are new to us but was already known thousands of years ago.

Let us see what the Makers Handbook has to say about the matter of eating fat. Particularly that thick fat layer that decorates the beef cut for the grill.

Eating of fat forbidden by God:
The Bible is still the truth and an amazing book of science. Bible and real Science agree We have already mentioned the fact that God instructed Noah to take seven couples of the clean animals into the ark, which tells us that Noah was already practicing the eating of —clean animals‖ for he knew of which he had to take seven pairs. So, it is not at all a new command given to General Mozes in Leviticus 3:17 It shall be a perpetual statute throughout your generations in all your dwellings, that ye shall eat neither fat nor blood. It is sometimes necessary for us to be instructed over and over again before it penetrates our thick sculls, so He repeats in Leviticus 7:22 And Yahweh spake unto Moses, saying, Leviticus 7:23 Speak unto the children of Israel, saying, Ye shall eat no fat, of ox, or sheep, or goat.
What I have stated here is general knowledge from abundance seen on the web. I am just flabbergasted that we as Christians will always seek from New Testament writings some scripture to justify our contraventions of the beautiful and good laws of the Almighty God; so did our first parents. But know this; when God says —No‖ it is —No‖. <u>The bible never contradicts itself. His Word is forever settled in Heaven.</u>
In our grocery stores one can find some excellent fatty stuff like Smart Balance and the very healthy Olive oil. I even prefer Smart Balance to butter. And that reminds me of what the butter said when it first met Smart Balance —I am not trying to look like you.‖ Tip: Spread avocado on a bagel instead of cream cheese. Use olive oil and garlic instead of whole milk and butter for a flavorful twist on mashed potatoes.
It always amazes me how quick people can find scripture to justify their disobedience, taking Bible texts completely out of context. When one tries to warn someone about contravening God's Law as written in the Old Testament, he or she might say

—Ah that is Old Testamentl. And with that they rest their case and continue in their disobedience; little do they care that by disregarding the Old Testament, you just don't have a New Testament:

This has everything to do with modern medicine:

The unity of Old and the New Testaments

The Bible says of itself: 2 Timothy 3:15 And that from a babe thou hast known the sacred writings which are able to make thee wise unto salvation through faith which is in Yahshua the Messiah. And further Psalms 19:8 the precepts of Yahweh are right, rejoicing the heart: The commandment of Yahweh is pure, enlightening the eyes. The Hebrew Script: Psalms 19:8 (19:9 in Heb.) Piquwdeey Yahweh yshaariym msamcheey- leeb mitsw Yahwehbaaraah m'iyrat `eeynaayim.

They are each other's counterparts. It is imperative that we rightly settle in our minds as to what position Messiah and His Apostles and the early Church took as regards to the Old Testament, so as to prevent us from butchering Scripture and by so doing hurting ourselves and cause us to be right out miserable. The Old Testament is God's truth enfolded--in the New it is unfolded to the Messianic nations [The Church]. In the Old Testament, events are predicted in the New they are [or ultimately will be] fulfilled. In the Old, even though it was Messiah involved in creation and discussions with people like Moses, Abraham, Joshua and others, He is concealed--in the New He is revealed, not only to certain individuals, but to all His Sheep. The Old is the root--the New is the branch· The Old is the bud --the New is the flower. The New Testament is impossible without the Old, as impossible as leaves and grapes without the branch and vine. One is the counterpart of the other; both are incomplete without the other.

A stern warning directly from the Word; Deuteronomy 4:2 Ye shall not add unto the word which I command you, neither shall ye diminish from it, that ye may keep the commandments of Yahweh your God which I command you. Yup, I know, Mozes did speak in the Hebrew tongue and so did the angel Gabriel to Mary.l Deuteronomy 4:2 Lo' tocipuw `al-hadaabaar 'sher 'aanokiy mtsaweh 'etkem wlo' tigr`uw mimenuwlishmor 'etmitswot Yahweh 'Eloheeykem 'sher 'aanokiy mtsaweh'etkem. {Hebrew]

The true Messiah of the New Testament is the YAHWEH of the Old, incarnate. In the burning bush Elohim said to Moses, "Say unto them 'I AM' [Yahweh] hath sent me unto you. "Yahshua [Simply means Yah the Savior] said, "Before Abraham was Yahweh or as it is written, I AM. This is His correct Name; not I was or I shall be, but the Great Everlasting —I AM. I get chills running down my back when I hear the Holy Name being butchered. That special night when the Angel Gabriel informed Miriam [Mary] that she will be instrumental to the incarnation of the Messiah, I am positively sure that he would have spoken to her in her own language when he said —Ye shall call His Name Yahshua, for it is He who shall save His people from their sin. He is the great I AM and He is the Great Yahshua. The Name means Yah the Savior or then Yahweh the Savior. When He eventually rode on that royal ass or donkey into Jerusalem He became very emotional and called out: Matthew 23:37 O Jerusalem, Jerusalem, thou that killest the prophets, and stonest them which are sent unto thee, how often would I have gathered thy children together, even as a hen gathereth her chickens under her wings, and ye would not! Messiah is the personification, the express image of God the Father: Hebrews 1:1-3 Who being the brightness of his glory, and the express image of his person, and upholding all things by the word of his power, when he had by himself purged our sins, sat down on the right hand of the Majesty on high; God revealed Himself through the spoken Word on Mount Sinai in the Old Testament and in the incarnate living Word on Mount Calvary in the New: John 1:1 In the beginning was the Word, and the Word was with God, and the Word was God. 2. The same was in the beginning with God. 3. All things were made by him; and without him was not any thing made that was made. Not only do we see Him here as the Messiah and God, but also as the Creator of everything. Just one more: Revelation 19:16 And he hath on his garment and on his thigh a name written, KING OF KINGS, AND LORD OF LORDS.

94

Let us bear in mind that Yahshua the Messiah was the Lord that dealt with man from Eden to the end. HE is the One that framed the LAW from the inset of creation; therefore it is ridiculous to assert that He would violate his own Laws. In Matthew 5:I7-I9 Yahshua said He "came not to destroy the law, but to fulfill" that it might be fulfilled in us who believe on Him. Instead of minimizing the law, Yahshua actually magnified the law as revealed in this passage in Matthew 5, He fulfilled all the law perfectly or He could not have been the transgressor's substitute and sin offering Isaiah 53: 11-12 He shall see of the travail of his soul, and shall be satisfied: by his knowledge shall my righteous servant justify many; for he shall bear their iniquities. 12. Therefore will I divide him a portion with the great, and he shall divide the spoil with the strong; because he hath poured out his soul unto death: and he was numbered with the transgressors; and he bare the sin of many, and made intercession for the transgressors.

It was Passover morning in 1977 when my wife and I in the company of Mr. And Mrs. Pat Boone stood there looking onto that rock formation of Golgotha; I could not help but to remark the fact that the place was true to its name, since it depicts a perfect skull. Why Golgotha? Calvary? It was our violation of these COMMANDMENTS that temporarily blotted out the "Sun of Righteousness" Malachi 3:2 But who may abide the day of his coming? And who shall stand when he appeareth? For he is like a refiner's fire, and like fullers' soap: from heaven; that sent Him to a dark Gethsemane, symbolized by the three hours of "darkness over all the earth" at His crucifixion Luke 23:44-45 And it was about the sixth hour, and there was a darkness over all the earth until the ninth hour. 45. And the sun was darkened, and the veil of the temple was rent in the midst. He hung between heaven and earth as forsaken of God and man, to pay the death penalty for our transgression, dying the death of a hated criminal. His very soul was poured out as our sin offering [Isaiah 53:II, 12]. Dare we imply by argument or lifestyle that He did this that we might transgress the laws of the Moral Governor of the Universe with impunity? On the contrary this, the greatest event of all history, was displaying God's evaluation of the law to the whole world, showing the awful penalty of its transgression, and the tremendous price of man's redemption. The Cross made our trespasses become exceedingly sinful, and should drive us to yielding ourselves unto confession, "that the righteousness of the law might be fulfilled in us, who walk not after the flesh but after the Spirit" Romans 8:4 That the righteousness of the law might be fulfilled in us, who walk not after the flesh, but after the Spirit. Deuteronomy 27:1 And Moses with the elders of Israel commanded the people, saying, Keep all the commandments which I command you this day.

The apostle Paul regarded the law of God seriously when he reminds us that ordinances are not the most important "but the keeping of the commandments of God" I Corinthians 7:19 Circumcision is nothing, and uncircumcision is nothing, but the keeping of the commandments of God. And in Romans 7:12 Wherefore the law is holy, and the commandment holy, and just, and It is for our benefit and blessing. Paul, before Felix, declared: "This I confess unto thee that after the way which they call heresy, so worship I the God of my fathers BELIEVING ALL THINGS WHICH ARE WRITTEN IN THE LAW and in the prophets" Acts 24:14 But this I confess unto thee, that after the way which they call heresy, so worship I the God of my fathers, believing all things which are written in the law and in the prophets:

I think that Christians [Messianics] would be smart to revert to the specifications of the New Covenant and rely not on our own understanding and our own feeble strength, but on the power and teaching of our Master Teacher, the Holy Spirit God. Yahshua said that the Holy Spirit would teach us in all things.. In the book of Hebrews, the Apostle declares what the New Covenant [Testament] really is, and he quotes from the prophet Jeremiah 31: 31-34 where our King and Lord proclaims: 31 Behold, the days come, saith the Lord, that I will make a new covenant with the house of Israel, and with the house of Judah: 32. Not according to the covenant that I made with their fathers in the day that I took them by the hand to bring them out of the land of Egypt; which my covenant they brake, although I was an husband unto them, saith the Lord: 33. But this shall be the covenant that I will make with the house of Israel; After those days, saith the Lord, I will put my law in their inward parts, and write it in their hearts; and will be their God, and they shall be my people. 34. And they shall teach no more every man his neighbor, and every man his brother, saying, Know the Lord: for they shall all know me, from the least of them unto the greatest of them, saith the Lord: for I will forgive their iniquity, and I will remember their sin no more.

The Apostle John speaks to us in this regard: "And hereby we know that we know him if we keep his commandments. He that saith 'I know him' and keepeth not his commandments is a liar and the truth is not in him" I John 2:3,4. And again, "And whatsoever we ask we receive of him because we keep his commandments and do those things that are pleasing in his sight" I John 3:22. "By this we know that we love the children of God when we love God and keep his commandments. For this is the love of God that we keep his commandments and his commandments are not grievous"

There is a terrible misnomer causing so many other misnomers, and that is the word —Jew‖. The very first time that this word was stuck to any part of the nations of Israel was at least one hundred and forty five years after the northern Tribes dispersed, primarily over Western Europe. They were despised by the south and were referred to as the —Scattered nations‖ which in the English is referred to as —Gentiles‖ meaning the genetic family. They were also referred to as the dispersed John 7:35 Then said the Jews among themselves, whither will he go, that we shall not find him? Will he go unto the dispersed among the Nations, and teach the Gentiles?. Please do not confuse the lost sheep with the title of heathen or pagan and do not call them Jews because they were no Jews. The nick name —Jew‖ or more correctly:‖Jud‖ were in fact only so dubbed on those peasants and farmers of Judah and Benjamin that remained in Judah during the Babylonian captivity, like Mordechai, the uncle of Ester who told them in Babylon that he was a Jud or Jew then. The other fact is that the Juds intermarried with the Idumeans, Esau's descendants, today, the Palestinians. They were the ones that produced the Harrods and, also, Pontius Pilot. Messiah called them "Generation of vipers" and so did John the Baptist. These are the crowd that was in control of the Temple order at the time of Yahshua [Jesus]. Read Matthew 10:5 These twelve Yahshua sent forth, and charged them, saying, Go not into any way of the Heathen, and enter not into any city of the Samaritans. 6. But go rather to the lost sheep of the house of Israel. So, who is the Church? The answer is simple: it is the one who believes, and who is that? It is he or she into whose heart has been put the Law and the Spirit. That is the Elect of the new Covenant. That is supreme Grace. —It is not every one that says Lord, Lord‖ What you witness in the land Israel today is not the return of the greater Israel but merely Jews that do not even believe in Yahshua as the Messiah; see Revelation 3:9 Behold, I will make them of the synagogue of Satan, which say they are Jews.

I quote the above Scripture that calls on you dear Christian not to ignore or spin Yahweh's holy Laws. The Almighty even promises to bless you richly if you obey His wonderful, beautiful ordinances. In fact, Scripture also says that if you don't, even your prayers are sin.

Dear reader, I even believe that the Bible as a whole is the Law of Yahweh the living Elohim. Just consider that day when —Ezra read the Law‖, the people remained standing half a day. Will you? Nehemiah 8:1 And all the people gathered themselves together as one man into the broad place that was before the water gate; and they spake unto Ezra the scribe to bring the book of the law of Moses, which Yahweh had commanded to Israel. 2. And Ezra the priest brought the law before the congregation, both of men and women, and all that could hear with understanding, upon the first day of the seventh month. 3. And he read therein before the street that was before the water gate from the morning until midday, before the men and the women, and those that could understand; and the ears of all the people were attentive unto the book of the law.

The Law Book contains The Ten Big Commandments on which is based all the laws and statutes and ordinances.. They are there, not for us to pick and choose, but to reverently be obeyed. The Almighty Father and Creator gave them all to us for our own good and for His glory. Deuteronomy 27:1 And Moses and the elders of Israel commanded the people, saying, Keep all the commandments which I command you this day.

In case you do not know that a command is more powerful than a law or a statute; a command is to be obeyed to the finest detail and is not optional. It is a military term and the contravention of it could mean death penalty. A law could be amended by decree but not a command..

A famous Bible text in our time that is often misquoted to suit the occasion is in Exodus 15 of which only the second part of the sentence is quoted namely —for I am the Lord that healeth thee‖. Deliberately your part of the bargain is omitted, as if you have no obligation toward The Almighty. While it is very true that no healing without God can occur, no not even an aspirin can cure your headache without the healing power of the Holy Spirit. But, now let us see what Scripture actually states: Exodus 15:26 and he said, If thou wilt diligently hearken to the voice of Yahweh thy God, and wilt do that which is right in his eyes, and wilt give ear to his commandments, and keep all his statutes, I will put none of the diseases upon thee, which I have put upon the Egyptians: for I am Yahweh that healeth thee. He did say —ALL!‖

We are to study ourselves thoroughly in the Word so as to be good ambassadors for King Messiah so as not to be ashamed. I remember one day, I was still very young, a sermon from my pastor on the reformation of the Church, where he emphasized the importance of a continuation of reformation. I remember how he repeated and exclaimed —Keep on keeping on reforming all the time."

It is God the Holy Spirit working in us to will and to work according to His good pleasure. It is a very dangerous thing when we get to the point where we think ourselves as know-alls. As a scholar of the Holy Scriptures, I am obligated to share with others that what He reveals to me from time to time. Things that we have cherished for so long are quite often the truth told in a funny way. I have learned over the years that the more I get to know, I also get to know how little I know. The Bible says, —My people are going astray because of a lack of knowledge.‖ I don't mind being called an ignoramus as long as I know that what I believe is unadulterated and Scriptural. We are to remember that the Word of Yahweh is alive and talks to us when reading; we must just listen like the wise old owl:

A wise old owl was perching on top of an oak
The more he saw, the less he spoke
The less he spoke the more he heard
Why can we not be like this wise old bird.

In the days when our Roman brethren were not allowed to eat meat on Fridays, a man was cooking a porky when he saw the priest coming; he grabbed the piggy by his hind legs, lifted it out of the pot and said —Some call you a pig, others call you a hog, but today I baptize you a fish.‖

Was that piggy sanctified in the New Testament?

As a child of Elohim I am obligated to share with my fellow believers that which the Holy Spirit teaches me. If I don't, their blood might just be claimed from my hands. Scripture says that it is an awful thing to fall in the hands of the Living God. Ezekiel 3:17 Son of man, I have made thee a watchman unto the house of Israel: therefore hear the word at my mouth, and give them warning from me. 18. When I say unto the wicked, Thou shalt surely die; and thou givest him not warning, nor speakest to warn the wicked from his wicked way, to save his life; the same wicked man shall die in his iniquity; but his blood will I require at thine hand.

19. Yet if thou warn the wicked, and he turn not from his wickedness, nor from his wicked way, he shall die in his iniquity; but thou hast delivered thy soul.

20. Again, When a righteous man doth turn from his righteousness, and commit iniquity, and I lay a stumbling block before him, he shall die: because thou hast not given him warning, he shall die in his sin, and his righteousness which he hath done shall not be remembered; but his blood will I require at thine hand.

21. Nevertheless if thou warn the righteous man, that the righteous sin not, and he doth not sin, he shall surely live, because he is warned; also thou hast delivered thy soul.

The warning is clear.

Faith is not for all men. John 10:26 But ye believe not, because ye are not of my sheep, as I said unto you.

10:27 My sheep hear my voice, and I know them, and they follow me:

10:28 And I give unto them eternal life; and they shall never perish; neither shall any man pluck them out of my hand. 2 Thes. 3:2 And that we may be delivered from unreasonable and wicked men: for all men have not faith.

3:3 But 𝓱𝓸𝓻is faithful, who shall e stablish you, and keep you from evil.

Great Doctors

I believe that doctors and nurses are a gift from Yahweh to us; they devote all their time to us, so much so that they sometimes do not have a normal family life; so let us appreciate them and remember them in our devotions.

It was just this past week that my cardiologist friend asked me to pray for him, as he was rather distracted. He is one of the kindest soft-spoken men I know. He is a devout Christian and an active member of his congregation, a great family man and wanting nothing except prayer. It gives me joy to mention his name every morning to my Heavenly Father, together with all the doctors whom I know as well as them that I have never met. We, as the children of Messiah, are obligated to pray for those gifted men. No doubt they are gifted indeed but remember they are human with limited abilities like everyone else; Therefore we aught to always pray for our pastors and schoolteachers. If you do not pray for them then you have no right to complain about them. No preacher can be successful in his sermon preparation unless his congregation supports him with prayers.

We owe gratitude to the Almighty for great doctors that unselfishly devote their lives to the medical profession for our welfare.

It was in 1952, when my lifelong friend graduated from medical school. To describe that occasion leaves me short of words; however, I can state that it was a solemn occasion with those new doctors taking the —Hippocratic Oath‖, written by Hypocrites circa 500 BC. This oath had from time to time been revised to match a variety of faiths. However it all boils down to one thing and that is that God given life is to be considered sacred.

I took liberty in copying that excellent old document: -

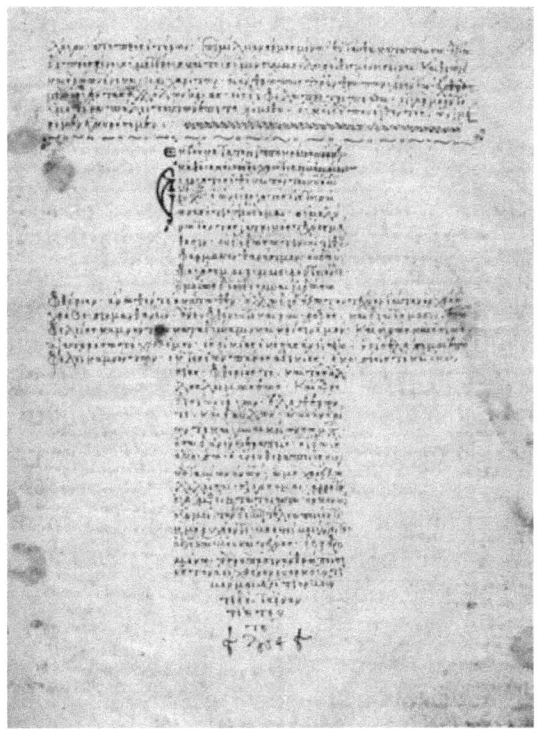

THE HIPPOCRATIC OATH

I SWEAR in the presence of the Almighty and before my family, my teachers and my peers that according to my ability and judgment I will keep this Oath and Stipulation.

TO RECKON all who have taught me this art equally dear to me as my parents and in the same spirit and dedication to impart knowledge of the art of medicine to others. I will continue with diligence to keep abreast of advances in medicine. I will treat without exception all who seek my ministrations, so long as the treatment of others is not compromised thereby and I will seek the counsel of particularly skilled physicians where indicated for the benefit of my patient.] How beautiful.]

I WILL FOLLOW that method of treatment, which according to my ability and judgment, I consider for the benefit of my patient and abstain from whatever, is harmful or mischievous. I will neither prescribe nor administer a lethal dose of medicine to any patient even if asked nor counsel any such thing nor perform the utmost respect for every human life from fertilization to natural death and reject abortion that deliberately takes a unique human life.

WITH PURITY, HOLINESS AND BENEFICENCE I will pass my life and practice my art. Except for the prudent correction of an imminent danger, I will neither treat any patient nor carry out any research on any human being without the valid informed consent of the subject or the appropriate legal protector thereof, understanding that research must have as its purpose the furtherance of the health of that individual. Into whatever patient setting I enter, I will go for the benefit of the sick and will abstain from every voluntary act of mischief or corruption and further from the seduction of any patient.

WHATEVER IN CONNECTION with my professional practice or not in connection with it I may see or hear in the lives of my patients which ought not be spoken abroad, I will not divulge, reckoning that all such should be kept secret.

WHILE I CONTINUE to keep this Oath inviolate may it be granted to me to enjoy life and the practice of the art and science of medicine with the blessing of the Almighty and respected by my peers and society, but should I trespass and violate this Oath, may the reverse by my lot.

When that Amen sounded, believe me dear reader, there were several well-lubricated eyes and nose sniffs.

A copy of this oath that decorated the wall in a beautiful gold frame of my late friend's office from the day he started practicing medicine until his death, after having lived up to that oath to the finest detail for over fifty years. I cherish his memory. At his graveside even the hardest men shed their tears.

I quote Hypocrites —Extreme remedies are very appropriate for extreme diseases.‖

I still think that some people talk too much about too many things that they know too little about. I know; I do. Cobus.

The stethoscope

Who does not remember the first time you saw the doc with little black pipes connected to his ears? And when the loveable old doc put that shiny end to the chest and moved it from one position to the other and the baby started crying and he took it off and gave it to the child to play with, and the little human immediately stopped the noise?

If you want to hear the story behind the beginning of this indispensable instrument where without a doctor will virtually be helpless in diagnosing a patient, well, I have searched the answer for you.

In the good old days when doctors had good bedside manners and great respect for a lady; you see, in those days almost all women were ladies, it happened one day that a gentleman doctor needed to examine a young woman; [he was doctor Laennec] hesitated to put his head to her chest. Ere this period, the doc had to put his ear on the body, where now he can move the sensor around beneath the clothing and not expose the vital statistics.

He then remembered a little incident that intrigued him when one day he took a hairpin and scraped one end of a plank while putting his ear to the other end. He thought of trying this principle of sound transmission. He rolled a few sheets of paper into a cylinder, pressed one end to the patient's chest, and held his ear to the other end. He wrote in his diary, "I was surprised and pleased to hear the beating of the heart much more clearly than if I had applied my ear directly to the chest."Thus, Dr.René-Théophile-Hyacinthe Laennec invented the stethoscope in France in 1816. It consisted of a wooden tube and was monaural. His device was similar to the common ear trumpet; indeed, his invention was almost indistinguishable in structure and function from the trumpet, which was commonly called a "microphone."

In 1850, George Camman substituted rubber for stiffer materials and made a more comfortable model—the forerunner of today's stethoscopes.

In 1851 Arthur Leared invented a binaural stethoscope, and in 1852 George Camman perfected the design of the instrument for commercial production, which has become the standard ever since. Camman also authored a major treatise on diagnosis by auscultation, which the refined binaural stethoscope made possible. By 1873, there were descriptions of a differential stethoscope that could connect to slightly different locations to create a slight stereo effect, though this did not become a standard tool in clinical practice.

Rappaport and Sprague designed a new stethoscope in the 1940's, which became the standard by which other stethoscopes are measured. Hewlett-Packard, later Philips, and today there are still cardiologists who consider it to be the finest acoustic stethoscope later made the Rappaport-Sprague. [Citation needed] Several other minor refinements were made to stethoscopes until in the early 1960's Dr. Littmann, a Harvard Medical School professor, created a new stethoscope that was lighter than previous models.

What are the sounds that a stethoscope reveals?

A normal heartbeat makes a lob-dup sound. This sound is created when the heart tissue vibrates when blood is thrown into turbulent oscillations as it is pushed against the heart valves and bounces back.

For 82 years I enjoyed excellent health for which I am profoundly grateful. But as the saying goes, good things don't last forever. Having had an extremely active business and professional life that invariably brought stress with it, I have put a heavy load on my blood pump with some requirement from the heart we may call —pay back.‖ How I thank Yahweh for those modern inventions that helped me making that —Pay back‖ and I thank our Creator for providing doctors that devote their lives to the welfare of mankind.

My heart is not a member of the cardio vascular labor union, but it went in a murmuring strike what they call atrial fibrillation. In asking what on earth is this atrial fib, the answer came simply and straight forward: —A variety of heart conditions can change the shape of heart valves or chambers and cause abnormal sounds. If the valves don't close completely, for example, some blood leaks back through the valve, making a whooshing, rasping, or blowing sound called a murmur.‖ It reminds me of an open water tap with water gushing out and then being shut of instantly gives you the sound of a water hammer.

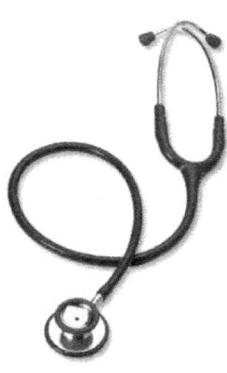 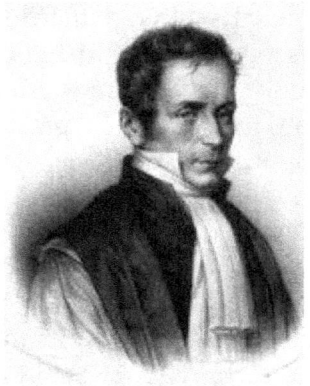

Thus Dr.René-Théophile-Hyacinthe Laennec invented the stethoscope in France in 1816

Blood Pressure Monitor

It was a Russian surgeon by name Nikolai Korotkoff who in 1905 developed the modern technique of using the stethoscope to listen for the sounds of blood flowing through the artery. This method proved to be extremely accurate and led to the discovery of hypertension.

What is blood pressure?

Blood pressure is the force exerted by the blood on blood vessel walls. Today, it's measured in millimeters of mercury, units that refer to the height to which a column of mercury is raised by an equivalent pressure.

Although physiologists who studied animals knew about the phenomenon of blood pressure in the 1700s, it was many years before physicians figured out how to measure it in humans. As soon as doctors had an accurate device and a simple procedure for measuring blood pressure, it became a normal part of a medical exam. Physicians could detect and monitor blood pressure over time, and they soon discovered hypertension, or chronic high blood pressure, a widespread and life-threatening condition.

Unfortunately, doctors had few options for treating hypertension and little understanding of its causes. Sometimes kidney disease was associated with hypertension, but in most cases, no cause could be identified.

It was not until 1901, after many trials and errors, that a suitable working partner for the Stethoscope was developed. It was the forerunner of the blood pressure monitor that intrigued me so much that I acquired one for the regular monitoring of our blood pressure.

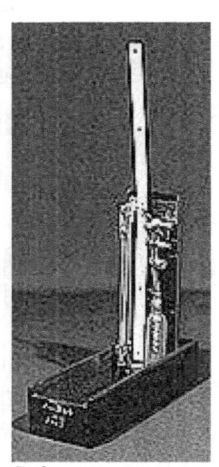

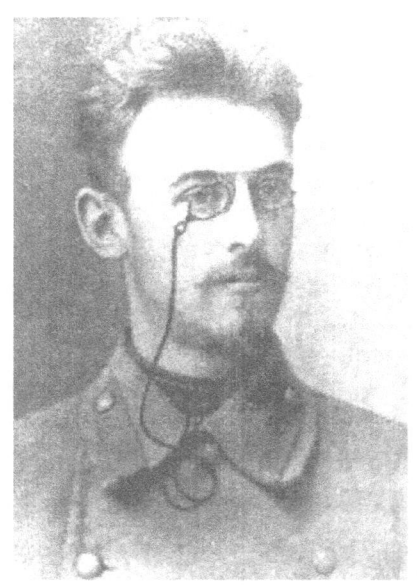

Sphygmomanometer
Russian Surgeon
Nikolai Korotkoff
1874 – 14 March 1920

Nikolai Korotkoff 1920 invented the mercury sphygmomanometer. All the time, all over the world, blood pressure readings are taken together with the listening of the —Korotkoff sounds‖ of heartbeats, thump-thump, thump thump through the earpieces of Laennec' S invention.

If we had to accredit someone with the invention of the blood pressure monitor, or responsible for it, it will without question be the Russian, Dr. Nicolai Korotkoff.

EKG/ECG

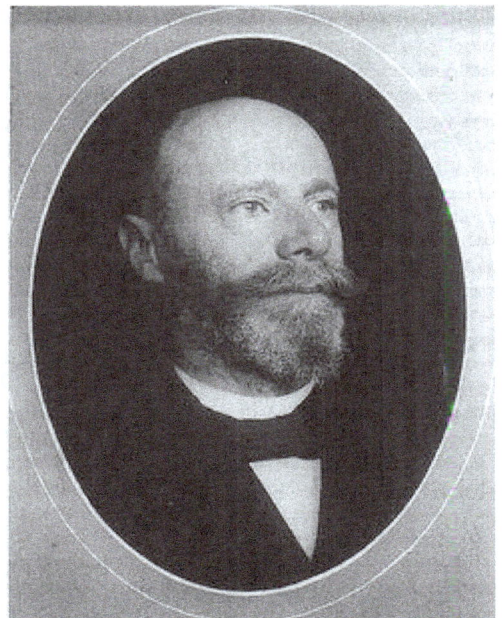

The inventor of the EKG, Willem Einthoven

As an electrical engineer, the Electro-Cardiogram was a fascination when I saw it for the first time in operation. I asked my physician friend to explain this intriguing little creation to me. He smiled and said —The Hollanders not only tamed the Cape of Storms, but invented many things for our use. Do you still love Ludwig van Beethoven? I know that you are crazy about his Fifth.‖

It happened in 1957 after an episode one night in the —Rohr gebiet‖ in Germany whilst there on business. Waking up at about midnight with the most excruciating chest pain, I thought it was a heart attack. What exasperated the situation was that I was six thousand miles from home. I went down to the lobby where there was only a night watch, a man who had no advice for me. As a Christian I just prayed that our Heavenly Father be merciful. I felt normal again after a few moments and went to sleep. The next day I proceeded to my destination in Hanover.

It was not until many months later that I experienced a recurrence and called my doctor friend James, who and without hesitation came over to my office, and took me in his car with windows down, up in the mountains for cool fresh air. Again the pain subsided. Immaterial of the fact that the attack ended, he sent me the very next day to Dr, Sadie in Johannesburg. The old cardiologist's diagnosis was, —This man will never die from a heart attack, and he has a heart like an ox. He will benefit by reducing his weight by a few pounds. It seems to me that his esophagus relaxes allowing stomach acids flowing up, to cause the pain.‖ Thanks to good old doctors and their use of the EKG. And of course a big thanks to that other Dutchman, Sir Doctor Enthoven, inventor of that machime.

It should be noted that sometimes it is abreviated ECG [Electrocardiogram], but EKG [Dutch/Afrikaans and German spelling Elektro-Kardio-Gram] seems to have stuck as more popular. Anyway, scientists have known for over 120 years that the heart gives off electrical currents when it beats, but it was the Dutch scientist Willem Enthoven who in the early 20th century discovered the nature of this phenomenon and who developed the electrocardiogram as a tool to look at the electrical conduction of the heart.   It has been a staple of diagnostic cardiovascular medicine since then.   The basic tracing used has changed little in decades, although the sophistication of the recording devices and the computer algorithms for automated interpretation have made dramatic changes in the last 20 years.

Dr. Willem Einthoven was born on May 21, 1860, in Semarang on the island of Java, in the former Dutch East Indies (now Indonesia). His father was Jacob Einthoven, born and educated in Groningen, The Netherlands, and an army medical officer in the Indies, who later became parish doctor in Semarang. His mother was Louise M.M.C. de Vogel, daughter of the then Director of

Finance in the Indies. Willem was the eldest son, and the third child in a family of three daughters and three sons.

At the age of six, Einthoven lost his father. Four years later his mother decided to return with her six children to Holland, where the family settled in Utrecht.

After having passed the "Hogere Burgerschool" (secondary school), he in 1878 entered the University of Utrecht as a medical student, intending to follow in his father's footsteps. His exceptional abilities, however, began to develop in quite a different direction. After being assistant to the ophthalmologist H. Snellen Sr. in the renowned eye-hospital "Gasthuis voor Ooglidders", he made two investigations, both of which attracted widespread interest. The first was carried out after Einthoven had gained his "candidaat" diploma (approximately equivalent to the B.Sc. degree), under the direction of the anatomist W. Koster, and was entitled "Quelques remarques sur le mécanisme de l'articulation du coude" (Some remarks on the elbow joint). Later he worked in close association with the great physiologist F.C. Donders, under whose guidance he undertook his second study, which was published in 1885 as his doctor's thesis: "Stereoscopie door kleurverschil." (Stereoscopy by means of colour variation) - one of Einthoven's teachers was the physicist C.H.D. Buys Ballot, who discovered the well-known law in meteorology.

That same year, 1885, he was appointed successor to A. Heynsius, Professor of Physiology at the University of Leiden, which he took up after having qualified as general practitioner in January 1886. His inaugural address was entitled "De leer der specifieke energieen" (The theory of specific energies). His first important research in Leiden was published in 1892: "Über die Wirkung der Bronchialmuskeln nach einer neuen Methode untersucht, und über Asthma nervosum" (On the function of the bronchial muscles investigated by a new method, and on nervous asthma), a study of great merit, mentioned as "a great work" in Nagel's "Handbuch der Physiologie". At that time he also began research into optics, the study of which occupied him ever since.

Some publications in this field were: "Eine einfache physiologische Erklärung für verschiedene geometrisch-optische Täuschungen" (A simple physiological explanation for various geometric-optical illusions) in 1898; "Die Accomodation des menschlichen Auges" (The accomodation of the human eye) in 1902; "The form and magnitude of the electric response of the eye to stimulation by light at various intensities", with W.A. Jolly in 1908.

Up till now, his talents had not yet been developed to the full. This opportunity came when he began the task of registering accurately the heart sounds, using a capillary electrometer. With this in view, he investigated the theoretical principles of this instrument, and devised methods of obtaining the necessary stability, and of correcting mathematically the errors in the photographically registered results due to the inertia of the instrument. Having found these methods he decided to carry out a thorough analysis of A.D. Waller's electrocardiogram - a study which has remained classic in its field.

This investigation led Einthoven to intensify his research. To avoid complex mathematical corrections, he finally devised the string galvanometer, which did not involve these calculations. Although the principle in itself was obvious, and practical applications of it were made in other fields of study, the instrument had to be precisioned and refined to make it usable for physiologists, and this took three years of laborious work. As a result of this, a galvanometer was produced which could be used in medical science as well as in technology; an instrument which was incomparable in its adaptability and speed of adjustment.

He then, with P. Battaerd, took up the study of the heart sounds, followed by research into the retina currents with W.A. Jolly (begun earlier with H. K. de Haas). The electrocardiogram itself he studied in all its aspects with numerous pupils and with visiting scientists. It was this last research, which earned him the Nobel Prize in Physiology or Medicine for 1924. In addition to this the string galvanometer has proved of the highest value for

114

the study of the periphery and sympathetic nerves.

In the remaining years of his life, problems of acoustics and capacity studies came within the sphere of his interests. The construction of the string phonograph (1923) could be considered as a consequence of this.

Einthoven possessed the gift of being able to devote himself entirely to a particular field of study. (His genius was actually more orientated towards physics than physiology.) As a result he was able to make penetrating inquiries into almost any subject, which came, within the scope of his interests, and to carry out his work to its logical conclusion.

Einthoven was a great believer in physical education. In his student days he was a keen sportsman, repeatedly urging his comrades "not to let the body perish". (He was President of the Gymnastics and Fencing Union, and was one of the founders of the Utrecht Student Rowing Club.) His first study on the elbow joint resulted from a broken wrist suffered while pursuing one of his favorite sports, and during the somewhat involuntary confinement his interest was awakened in the pro- and supination movements of the hand and the functions of the shoulder and elbow joints.

The string galvanometer has led countless investigators to study the functions and diseases of the heart muscle. The laboratory at Leiden became a place of pilgrimage, visited by scientists from all over the world. For this, suffering mankind has much to owe to Einthoven. In electrocardiography the string galvanometer is the most reliable tool. Although it has been superseded by portable types and by models utilizing amplification techniques used in radio communication (Einthoven has always mistrusted the use of condensers, fearing the distortion of curves), cardiograms from the string galvanometer have remained the standard of reference in numerous cases to this day.

Einthoven was a member of the Dutch Royal Academy of

Sciences, the meetings of which he hardly ever missed. He frequently took part in the debates himself, and his sharp criticism frequently found weaknesses in many a lecture.

Einthoven married in 1886 Frédérique Jeanne Louise de Vogel, a cousin, and sister of Dr. W.Th. de Vogel, former Director of the Dienst der Volksgezondheid (Public Health Service) in the Dutch East Indies. There were four children: Augusta (b. 1887), who was married to R. Clevering, an engineer; Louise (b. 1889), married to J.A.R. Terlet, pastor emeritus; Willem (1893-1945) - a brilliant electro-technical engineer who was responsible for the development of the vacuum model of the string galvanometer and for its use in wireless communication, and who was Director of the Radio Laboratory in Bandung, Java; and Johanna (b. 1897), a physician.

He died on the 29th of September 1927, after long suffering.

As published in Les Prix Nobel.

Direct quote: **Cancer Update from Johns Hopkins**:

After years of the medical world telling people that chemotherapy is the only way to try [_Try' being the key word] to eliminate cancer, John's Hopkins is finally starting to tell you that there is an alternative way.   .

1. Every person has cancer cells in the body. These cancer cells do not show up in the standard tests until they have multiplied to a few billion. When doctors tell cancer patients that there are no more cancer cells in their bodies after treatment, it just means the tests are unable to detect the cancer cells because they have not reached the detectable size.

2. Cancer cells occur between 6 to more than 10 times in a person's lifetime.

3. When the person's immune system is strong the cancer cells will be destroyed and prevented from multiplying and forming tumors.

4. When a person has cancer it indicates the person has nutritional deficiencies. These could be due to genetic, environmental, food and lifestyle factors.

5. To overcome the multiple nutritional deficiencies, changing diet and including supplements will strengthen the immune system.

6. Chemotherapy involves poisoning the rapidly-growing cancer cells and also destroys rapidly-growing healthy cells in the bone marrow, gastrointestinal tract etc, and can cause organ damage, like liver, kidneys, heart, lungs etc.

7. Radiation while destroying cancer cells also burns, scars and damages healthy cells, tissues and organs.

8. Initial treatment with chemotherapy and radiation will often reduce tumor size. However prolonged use of chemotherapy and radiation do not result in more tumor destruction.

9. When the body has too much toxic burden from chemotherapy and radiation the immune system is either compromised or destroyed, hence the person can succumb to various kinds of infections and complications.

10. Chemotherapy and radiation can cause cancer cells to mutate and become resistant and difficult to destroy.
    Surgery can also cause cancer cells to spread to other sites.
11. An effective way to battle cancer is to starve the cancer cells by not feeding it with the foods it needs to multiply.

*CANCER CELLS FEED ON:

a. Sugar is a cancer-feeder. By cutting off sugar it cuts off one important food supply to the cancer cells. Sugar substitutes like NutraSweet, Equal, Spoonful, etc are made with Aspartame and it is harmful. A better natural substitute would be Manuka honey (a New Zealand Honey - can be found at some health food stores or online {*Amazon.com*}) or molasses, but only in very small amounts. Table salt has a chemical added to make it white in color Better alternative is Bragg's amino or sea salt.
b. Milk causes the body to produce mucus, especially in the gastro-intestinal tract. Cancer feeds on mucus. Cutting out milk and substituting with unsweetened soymilk cancer are starving cells.

   C. Cancer cells thrive in an acid environment. A meat-based diet is acidic and it is best to eat fish, and a little chicken rather than beef or pork. Meat also contains livestock antibiotics, growth hormones and parasites, which are all harmful, especially to people with cancer.

   D. A diet made of 80% fresh vegetables and juice, whole grains, seeds, nuts and a little fruits help put the body into an alkaline environment. About 20% can be from cooked food including beans. Fresh vegetable juices provide live enzymes that are easily absorbed and reach

118

down to cellular levels within 15 minutes to nourish and enhance growth of healthy cells. To obtain live enzymes for building healthy cells try and drink fresh vegetable juice (most vegetables including bean sprouts) and eat some raw vegetables 2 or 3 times a day. Enzymes are destroyed at temperatures of 104 degrees F (40 degrees C).

e. Avoid coffee, tea, and chocolate, which have high caffeine Green tea is a better alternative and has cancer-fighting properties. Water-best to drink purified water, or filtered, to avoid known toxins and heavy metals in tap water. Distilled water is acidic; avoid it.

12. Meat protein is difficult to digest and requires a lot of digestive enzymes. Undigested meat remaining in the intestines becomes putrefied and leads to more toxic buildup.

13. Cancer cell walls have a tough protein covering. By refraining from or eating less meat it frees more enzymes to attack the protein walls of cancer cells and allows the body's killer cells to destroy the cancer cells.

14. Some supplements build up the immune system (IP6, Florescence, Essiac, anti-oxidants, vitamins, minerals, EFAs etc.) to enable the body's own killer cells to destroy cancer cells. Other supplements like vitamin E are known to cause apoptosis, or programmed cell death, the body's normal method of disposing of damaged, unwanted, or unneeded cells.

15. Cancer is a disease of the mind, body, and spirit.

A proactive and positive spirit will help the cancer warrior be a survivor. Anger, un-forgiveness and bitterness put the body into a stressful and acidic environment. Learn to have a loving and forgiving spirit. Learn to relax and enjoy life life.

16. Cancer cells cannot thrive in an oxygenated

119

environment. <u>Exercising daily</u>, and <u>deep breathing</u> help to get more oxygen down to the cellular level. Oxygen therapy is another means employed to destroy cancer cells.

1. No plastic containers <u>in   microwave</u>.
2. No water bottles <u>in freezer</u>.
3. No plastic wrap <u>in   microwave</u>.

Johns Hopkins has recently sent this out in its newsletters. This information is being circulated at Walter Reed Army Medical Center as well. Dioxin chemicals cause cancer, especially breast cancer. <u>Dioxins are highly poisonous</u> to the cells of our bodies. Don't freeze your plastic bottles with water in them as this releases dioxins from the plastic. Recently, Dr Edward Fujimoto, Wellness Program Manager at Castle Hospital, was on a TV program to explain this health hazard. He talked about dioxins and how bad they are for us. He said that we should not be heating our food in the microwave using plastic containers. This especially applies to foods that contain fat. He said that the combination of fat, high heat, and plastics releases dioxin into the food and ultimately into the cells of the body. Instead, he recommends using glass, such as Corning Ware, Pyrex or ceramic containers for heating food. You get the same results, only without the dioxin. So such things as TV dinners, instant ramen and soups, etc., should be removed from the container and heated in something else. Paper isn't bad but you don't know what is in the paper. It's just safer to use tempered glass, Corning Ware, etc. He reminded us that a while ago some of the fast food restaurants moved away from the foam containers to paper. The dioxin problem is one of the   reasons.

Also, he pointed out that <u>plastic wrap, such as Saran</u>, is just as dangerous when placed over foods to be cooked in the microwave. As the food is nuked, the high heat causes poisonous toxins to actually melt out of the plastic wrap and drip into the food. Cover food with a paper towel instead.

How does the saying go? One ounce of prevention is better that a pound of cure; thus considering all that we learn from the written chapters, the oinks and other forbidden food, considering it comes to us from the Maker's Hand Book, why not try to prevent rather than try to cure when it is too late.

As a matter of interest, the Walter Reed Hospital is named after another great medical doctor that made the discovery that the yellow fever is caused by the bite of a disease-carrying mosquito, the anopheles. I still remember the days of old when we ever had the pyagra flit pump ready to fight off that irritating buzz of mosquitoes. As children we had to watch out for the malaria carrier, which was identified from other species by his sitting posture. Where his other namesakes sat in a flush position on the object, this mean chap sits in a diagonal manner.

The name Walter Reed Hospital is well known, so named after a great doctor, is the Walter Reed military Hospital.

Walter Reed

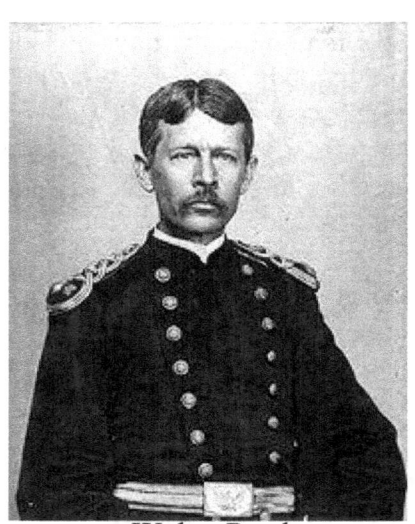

Walter Reed

Born	September 13, 1851 Belroi, Virginia USA.
Died	November 22, 1902 (aged 51) Washington D.C
Occupation	Military Physician
Spouse	Emilie Lawrence (m. 1876)

Aedes Aegypti Mosquito Information

Adult females lay their eggs in standing water, which can be a salt marsh, a lake, a puddle, a natural reservoir on a plant, or an artificial water container such as a plastic bucket. The first three stages are aquatic and last 5–14 days, depending on the species and the ambient temperature; eggs hatch to become larva, then pupae. The adult mosquito emerges from the pupa as it floats at the water surface. Adults live for 4–8 weeks. As a child, I spent many days playing under the fifty feet high eucalyptus trees behind our farm home. My parents had told me that the eucalyptus is the defense against mosquitoes.

Mosquitoes have mouthparts that are adapted for piercing the skin of plants and animals. While males typically feed on nectar and plant juices, the female needs to obtain nutrients from a "blood meal" before she can produce eggs.

There are about 3,500 species of mosquitoes found throughout the world. In some species of mosquito, the females feed on humans, and are therefore vectors for a number of infectious diseases affecting millions of people per year

The son of a Methodist minister, he became a United States Army officer about a decade after the conflict that had maimed his older brother for life.   Reed's conception of our nation embraced both the western and northern regions of our country and was perhaps similar to the notion of imperial destiny that Theodore Roosevelt espoused. Walter Reed's service at desolate Army outposts in hostile Indian territory included tours of duty not only in the Apache country of Arizona, but in the Sioux territory of the Dakotas where he treated survivors of the massacre at Wounded Knee. This was an age when their white countrymen often hated Native Americans. Reed fought for the improvement of reservation conditions in an era when these settlements were administered as death camps. Reed and his wife adopted an Indian child, a little girl. Reed's gallantry was further proven near the end of his career by his willingness to include him among the other human subjects infected with yellow fever in a test done in order to establish the disease's cause and stages. It is an accident of history that Reed was temporarily called back from Cuba to Washington in order to report on typhoid fever and was spared the ordeal of serving as a test subject. The other test subjects were men half his own age and better able to withstand the ensuing illness. One died. Reed survived and lived to record his findings that proved that yellow fever, much like malaria was transmitted by mosquitoes. This research, done in Cuba not long after the end of the Spanish-American War, helped physicians to understand and control the disease during a period when American troops were stationed in Cuba and was important later in the effort to construct the Panama Canal. Reed practiced medicine at a time when the microscope was becoming an important tool of medical research and he was fascinated by the study of microorganisms. Due to the fact that Walter Reed is popularly honored for his research of yellow fever it is often overlooked that he worked as part of a team that studied typhoid fever. His commitment to the ideal of scientific progress for the improvement of human life might strike the contemporary reader as an archaic ethic. One wonders what Walter Reed would have thought of a century in which medical science has become an instrument of death and suffering. Walter Reed's character was that of a courageous visionary whose strong sense of personal discipline required that he think and act in a humane manner in accordance with the Christian tradition, Walter Reed was born at the small country crossroads village of Belroi in Gloucester County, Virginia on September 13, 1851, Walter Reed was the fifth and last child born to Pharaba White Reed and her husband, Lemuel. The family home at Belroi is maintained today by the Association for the Preservation of Virginia Antiquities as a museum and contains many fascinating items from that time. Gloucester County honors Reed's memory with not only a hospital named after him but a new shopping center as well, one that features a big grocery store and a video rental shop. Like many other people residing in Gloucester County, I did not know very much about Reed's life when I began my bit of research. I wanted to learn something I thought I ought to already know.

James H. Bailey wrote about Walter Reed's birth and childhood in an article that appeared in the winter 1951 issue of the <u>Virginia Cavalcade</u>, a magazine published by the Virginia State Library at Richmond.   Bailey describes the setting and circumstances of Walter Reed's birth as follows... "The good folk of Gloucester County's Methodist congregation were disturbed. The parsonage had burned to the ground, and on any day the new circuit rider, the Reverend Lemuel Sutton Reed, would arrive from North Carolina with his wife, daughter, and three sons. To make the matter worse, rumor said that this already sizable family was about to be enlarged. The owner of Belroi Plantation saved the situation. Immediately he had his overseer move to a temporary shelter and turned that employee's quarters over to the clergyman and his family. Thus it happened that on September 13, 1851, Walter Reed, the father of modern public health, was born in a borrowed cabin consisting of two rooms and a garret.'

Lemuel Sutton Reed was a Methodist minister and his ministry took the family to a number of postings in Virginia and North Carolina. The Reeds resided in a number of small towns such as Gatesville, Murfreesboro and Farmville. Bailey's article in the <u>Virginia Cavalcade</u> describes Walter as an ordinary child whose behavior gave no hint of future greatness. "At Farmville, where his father served neighboring churches, six-year-old Walter began his education in a one-room school kept by a Mrs. Booker.   The child's appearance was very attractive, and his manners were noticeably gracious. A typical boy, he loved to roam the banks of the Appomattox and to watch the ox carts bringing in tobacco to the warehouses. Nothing about him would have led an observer to believe that this lads name would be chronicled with those of Lister and Pasteur. He gave not the slightest indication of any interest in science."

Walter's older brothers Tom and James both fought for the Confederacy and James, a Sergeant, lost a hand at the battle of Antietam but continued in active military duty. Dr. William Bean, a man awarded the status of professor emeritus at the University of Iowa's College of Medicine, studied the career of Walter Reed for many years and wrote what is considered to be the most authoritative biography of Reed's life. Like Reed, Bean took his MD degree at the University of Virginia and went on to serve in the Army Medical Corps. Bean saw action in the Pacific theater during the Second World War, according to the obituary recording his death in 1989 written by Alfred Soffer for the Journal of the American Medical Association. Bean's biography of Walter Reed was published in 1982. In this work, Bean records something of the widespread anguish and suffering the war brought to many Virginians by quoting from a diary kept by Walter's brother, James. The untold thousands of households experiencing similar tragic circumstances at the war's end might in the reader's mind, multiply the personal pain and heartbreak revealed in the following passage. "When I arrived home my father said to me: 'well, my son, it is all over now.' But I replied, 'No, sir: we will rest up awhile and then we will . . . lick them out of their boots.' But Alas! We never did." Bean also records that during 1864 while the Reed family resided at Lawrenceville, Walter and Christopher Reed attempted to hide their family's horses from the marauding cavalry of Union General Phil Sheridan. The boys were captured then released by the Federal troopers. At the war's end Lemuel Reed obtained a posting at Charlottesville, Virginia, in order that his sons might have the opportunity to attend the university in that town.

Howard Kelly's scholarly biography of Walter Reed was first copyrighted in 1906, only four years after the death of its subject. This entertaining work presents the life of a man as seen by a contemporary, a writer assessing a public figure by the contemporary standards of the time. Kelly's conversational narrative style seems casual in comparison with the intensely researched writing of Bean the historian. Kelly comments with admiration that Walter Reed was exceptionally young at the time he was admitted to the University's medical program. Kelly quotes a letter sent to him by Dr. A. R. Buckmaster, professor of obstetrics and practical medicine at the University of Virginia. The letter indicates Walter Reed's exceptional academic ability and strength of character, Personality traits that would enable him to complete his course of study at the university in half the time taken by most students. Buckmaster's letter, cited by Kelly, reads as follows. "Walter Reed was at the University of Virginia two sessions. In 1867 he took Latin, Greek, English literature, and another study in the academic department. In 1868 he studied medicine and was graduated after one year's work. This in itself shows that he was an unusual man. The standard was very high and no man could have reached it unless he were a very clever student...in earning his degree he proved himself above the average."

Bean comments about the intellectual climate at the University during these post-war years. "The faculty included such distinguished men as Basil Guildersleeve, the Greek professor who was to leave later for the new Johns Hopkins University: William McGuffey, the Presbyterian minister from Cincinnati who taught Moral Philosophy and wrote McGuffey's Reader; and William Wertenbacker, the librarian, who had known Mr. Jefferson well and who allowed Walter to use an alcove as a study." In addition to attending lectures medical students were expected to familiarize themselves with the human anatomy by dissecting the corpses of criminals and paupers. The school also sponsored a small outpatient-teaching clinic. Reed graduated third in his class and then traveled to New York where he continued his medical studies at Bellevue Hospital Medical College. Myra Gregory Knight echoes Bean's assessment of conditions at Bellevue Hospital in her review of Bean's biography of Walter Reed. Bellevue is described as being at that time, "the world's biggest, bloodiest and busiest hospital." Reed later worked at several hospitals located in Brooklyn. Biographers agree that Reed was astonished by the unsanitary conditions he encountered in the urban tenement slum districts of the city and saddened by the human misery these unhealthy conditions created.

Nina Page, an APVA volunteer working at the Walter Reed birthplace in Gloucester County, has written an unpublished paper about four pages long that summarizes material first presented in an article written for Stripe, a publication intended for patients and staff at Walter Reed Army Medical Center in Washington, D.C. Mrs. Page has served as Secretary for the Joseph Bryan Branch of the Association for the Preservation of Virginia Antiquities. This local chapter opens the Walter Reed home at Belroi each year on the Sunday closest to the anniversary of Reed's birthday, September 13th. Mrs. Page prepared her manuscript for use by the volunteer tour guides working at the house. Mrs. Page indicates that in 1874 Reed traveled south to visit his parents during which time he met his future wife, Emilie Lawrence of Murfreesboro, North Carolina. Mrs. Page notes, "In letters to her, he disclosed his intention to give up private practice and to apply for a commission as a medical officer in the Army where he reasoned that he would have a greater opportunity for research and more financial security. Walter and Emilie were married April 25th, 1875, in Murfreesboro."

After passing the required medical exams, Walter Reed was appointed an assistant surgeon in the United States Army on June 26th, 1875. His rank was that of first lieutenant. Lt. Reed spent the next five years in service at Ft. Lowell and Ft. Apache, Army posts located in Arizona. Reed's wife joined him at San Francisco in order to accompany him and make their home in what were often difficult surroundings. Bean comments, "Emilie's girlhood had been comfortable and sheltered. It was undoubtedly the most courageous act of her life when she took off from Virginia for San Francisco, surviving some kind of train wreck en route. It may well have been the bravest act of Walter Reed's life, which included many brave acts, for him to bring his wife to the Wild West. Perhaps the fierce mustache that he had grown during their separation, and wore when he met her in the Palace Hotel, was an unconscious gesture of self-protection on his part, for by now he knew that some of the 'horrors' of army life, as she girlishly called them, would be impossible to ignore. They met on November 5th, 'after six months of sighs and tears and protestations that no other human beings were ever so cruelly dealt with.' One salutes the tenacity and optimism of first love." Bean tells us that Walter and Emilie spent two weeks in San Francisco before making the 500-mile trip to Arizona. This journey took twenty-three days and was in all likelihood made in an army ambulance drawn by mules. The Reeds camped out at night in the wilderness. Spending many nights in terror and tears, Emilie would cry out for her husband whenever he moved out of sight. She would call, "Where are you Dr. Reed?" Reed wrote in a letter quoted by Bean that Emilie had shown great courage on this difficult trek. "I must give her credit for great bravery on this, her first night in an ambulance." Reed himself was daunted now by the difficulties ahead of them. "I'm afraid if there had been a stone wall nearby I should have brought my head in violent contact with it."

Many people of that era might perceive of the conditions in the far west of the North American continent to be hellish due to the trackless immensity of the hot dusty desert landscape. Temperatures at Camp Lowell near Tucson were reported at 115 degrees Fahrenheit in the shade. Mrs. Page writes that a son named Walter Lawrence Reed was born at Ft. Apache on December 4th, 1877. Reed was promoted to the rank of captain in 1880. Not long afterwards Reed was temporarily transferred to Ft. McHenry in Baltimore and then posted to Ft. Omaha, Nebraska. A daughter named Emilie Lawrence Reed was born at Ft. Omaha on July 12th, 1883. In October of that same year Walter Reed would assume duties as director of a military hospital located at Ft. Sidney, one of four military posts that had been established mainly to protect construction crews building the Union Pacific Railroad across the Great Plains in the late 1860's. Gordon Stelling Chappell describes the fort as it appeared during Walter Reed's time of service there in an article published about twenty-five years ago in the quarterly journal of the Nebraska State Historical Society. "The military post in the trans-Mississippi West bore little similarity to the stockaded forts protected by blockhouses portrayed in James Fenimore Cooper's fiction and the writings of Francis Parkman about a now long-past woodland frontier. Fort Sidney was typical among trans-Mississippi garrisons, consisting of a scattering of buildings set out on the prairie without semblance of fortified protection other than an ornamental picket fence. The central feature of the post was a vast parade ground, which the principal structures faced. Officers' quarters, which looked like ordinary Victorian civilian houses except that they were all alike, were on the west side. Facing them from across the parade were quartermaster and commissary storehouses and offices and the hospital. An infantry barracks stood on the north side, and on the south was a cavalry

129

barracks, with laundresses' quarters (for married enlisted men whose wives were laundresses) behind it. Behind these were the stables and blacksmith shop on the slope leading down to Lodgepole Creek. The buildings of the time were either of frame or 'concrete' (lime-grout) construction." Chappell's article includes a schematic diagram or plan of Fort Sidney dated 1871 that indicates the locations of several other important buildings such as the magazine, the guard house, a bakery, a carpenter's shop, an ice house, and a coal house, as well as a well. Chappell notes the grim conditions faced by Dr. Reed at Fort Sidney. Three years prior to Reed's posting, Lieutenant Colonel John Edward Summers, medical director of the Department of the Platte, had visited Ft. Sidney and written a report which stated that, — . . . the Hospital is shabbily constructed and very far from that which it was believed and hoped it would be." Chappell provides some insight into Walter Reed's initial reactions to conditions at Ft. Sidney. "Upon taking charge of medical affairs at Fort Sidney," Reed wrote in that official, calf-bound volume known as the Record of Medical History of Post, "I find the ward rather full of 'ugly' cases." Reed encountered numerous cases of typhoid fever at this isolated military outpost.

In 1890 Dr. Reed was assigned to Baltimore where he was given the duty of examining new recruits. While in Baltimore Dr. Reed studied bacteriology at the new Johns Hopkins Hospital. After completing studies at Johns Hopkins, Reed relocated his family to Washington, D.C. where he taught at the Army Medical School and served as curator of its museum. Bean writes, "He was forty-two when he became a professor, and had previously had no formal teaching experience. He was beginning to know for the first time the stimulation and excitement of kindling the minds of other men. It was a challenge to explore a complicated new subject, but it was equally a challenge to keep the attention of physicians--some of whom were present because of the army's orders rather than any interest of their own." Bean quotes from a letter written by one of Reed's students. "His lectures, beside satisfying the zealous seeker for knowledge, were spiced with humor . . . which made the relations between him and his students a freer and more sympathetic one. His language was always interesting . . . When he was at his best, his voice would reach a high falsetto note . . . due to his characteristic method of impressing important facts upon dull or indurate intellects. His students never feared him, but from the start regarded him with filial affection . . . He was constantly at the side of his pupils in the laboratory, advising, encouraging, counseling and, above all, instructing." It was at Johns Hopkins that Reed would first encounter James Carroll, an English workingman employed as a hospital steward. Carroll immigrated to America in 1874 and enlisted in the Army. As a sergeant serving at posts located in Minnesota and in Dakota Territory, Carroll decided to pursue a career in medicine. He attended medical lectures in St. Paul, Minnesota, and later at the City University of New York. He took his medical degree from the University of Maryland. For much of their professional lives Carroll was of great service to Reed, but Bean remarks that later in life and after Reed's death, Carroll would suffer from envy, feeling that he never received the credit that was rightfully due him for his part in Reed's medical research.

From 1891 to 1893 Reed was posted in the Dakotas. Dr. Bean's biography of Reed devotes some pages in describing this bleak period in Walter Reed's career. Yet it was in these primitive and often filthy conditions of frontier post life that Dr. Reed became the public health advocate of sanitary measures as a means of preventing infectious disease. Reed was promoted to the rank of major in 1893 and reassigned back east to Washington, D.C., where he served as curator of the Army Medical Museum (now part of the Armed Forces Institute of Pathology) and taught the subject of Clinical Microscopy at the Army Medical School (now known as the Walter Reed Army Institute of Research). Mrs. Page reports that Major Reed held a chair in bacteriology at the Columbian University, now known as George Washington University. Mrs. Page indicates the great number of papers published by Reed at this time concerning his original research. "Between 1892 and 1902 Reed published 27 papers on original work, encompassing a wide variety of subjects including; cholera, erysipelas, leukemia, malaria, pneumonia, typhoid, vaccinations and yellow fever."

Walter Reed was appointed as head of a board of medical officers investigating the spread of typhoid fever at a number of U.S. Army encampments in mid-August of 1898, just after the Spanish-American War. This board's findings indicated that the disease was spread to humans by flies that had contacted the bacilli in human excrement. Impure drinking water contaminated with these same bacilli was seen as another means by which the malady was spread. The success of this investigation brought about Dr. Reed's appointment in May of 1900 as director to a similar board of medical officers investigating the cause of yellow fever, another disease that plagued American Army bases, especially in tropical regions. James V. Writer, a free-lance author from Silver Spring, Maryland, writes about the disease in an article he wrote about Walter Reed for American History. "People called it yellow jack, for the flag raised by ships to warn that there was yellow fever aboard, and during the nineteenth century, it was 'simply the single most dreaded disease in the Americas.' In the United States, yellow fever came in the spring or summer and stayed until the first frost. Devastating yellow fever epidemics swept through many of America's Southern and East Coast port cities during the nation's early history. In the years between 1702 and 1800, the fever appeared roughly 35 times, with an epidemic in Philadelphia killing more than four thousand in 1793. An estimated half-million Americans contracted the fever between that year and the beginning of the twentieth century. About 100,000 victims succumbed to the disease during that period, 41,000 in New Orleans alone. The deadliest flare-up occurred along the Mississippi River, from the Gulf of Mexico to Memphis, Tennessee, in 1878. More than 20,000 people died that year as the fever swept upstream." Writer records the observations of Mathew Carey in an account of one outbreak in Philadelphia. "Many never walked on the footpath, but went into the middle of the streets, to avoid being infected by passing houses wherein people had died. Acquaintances and friends avoided each other in the streets, and only signified their regard with a cold nod. The old custom of shaking hands fell into such general disuse, that many were affronted at even the offer of a hand."

Writer defines yellow fever as, "an acute, infectious viral disease, with characteristics ranging from fever and flu-like symptoms in mild cases, to jaundice, internal bleeding, and liver and kidney damage in severe attacks." Writer indicates that the measures taken by the federal government to control yellow fever came about not because of a concern for American citizens as a matter of domestic policy, but rather as a wartime policy seeking to protect the health of American servicemen stationed in Cuba and other parts of the Caribbean during and shortly after the Spanish-American War. Writer notes, "American General Fitzhugh Lee, consul general to Cuba, said the scourge 'is worse than I ever knew it to be.' Meanwhile, at an American officers' mess of eight men, an old English toast was resurrected: 'to those who are gone already and here's to the next to go!' Six of the men were soon dead." The Army's surgeon general appointed a board to study yellow fever in Cuba and Dr. Walter Reed was named as director. The other members were James Carroll, Aristides Agramonte--a Cuban, and Jesse Lazear. Another talented physician, Dr. Henry Rose Carter, would later join them. Carter had studied yellow fever in the Mississippi Valley and concluded that an incubation period was required after the mosquito was first infected with yellow fever in order for the insect to be able to transmit the disease. Writer notes that the legacy of Reed's research would be seen in the work of Major William Crawford Gorgas, a sanitary and public health engineer stationed in Havana and a contemporary of Reed's who initially doubted Reed's theories. He was converted into an enthusiastic supporter. Of Gorgas Writer explains, "Once the mosquito hypothesis had been proven, it fell to then-Major William Crawford Gorgas to rid Havana of the life threatening pests. Later, his application in Panama of the lessons learned in Cuba made possible the long-dreamed-of construction of a canal connecting the Atlantic and Pacific oceans."

Dr. Joshua Nott of New Orleans had published a medical article that theorized that mosquitoes might be the agent of transfer for yellow fever in 1848. Dr. Carlos Juan Finlay of Cuba, a respected medical authority, was making the same assertion about this time, also. Reed came to the same conclusion after realizing that a prisoner in a guardhouse who came down with the illness could not have had many other opportunities for contact with the outside world other than the tiny insects that were able to fly through barred windows. Writer quotes from an article written years later by Reed and published in a medical journal. "It was conjectured at that time that, perhaps, some insect capable of conveying the infection, such as the mosquito had entered through the cell window, bitten this particular prisoner, and then passed out again." Yet the theory needed to be tested in controlled laboratory conditions. Dr. Jesse Lazear, a companion and associate of Dr. Reed, subjected himself to the bite of an infected insect and died. James Carroll repeated the experiment and became very ill. Reed would name the military camp soon established for the study of yellow fever after Dr. Lazear. Bean describes Dr. Jesse Lazear in the following passage. "In view of his later premature and tragic death, one cannot think of Lazear without great sadness. He was from all accounts a wonderfully agreeable man whose company gave Reed and the rest of them much pleasure. Agramonte, who had been Lazear's classmate in medical school, called him 'the type of the old southern gentleman, affectionate with a high sense of honor, a staunch friend and faithful.' Lazear had just joined the volunteer Army Medical Corps, having presented recommendations from William Welch himself. He was uneasily aware of being only thirty-three, but his background was formidable, including graduation in medicine from Columbia, an internship in Bellevue, work in pathology and bacteriology in Germany, and a teaching appointment at the Hopkins Hospital, where he worked under Osler and Thayer. As Thayer's junior associate, he had investigated the details of the newly discovered role of the mosquito in transmitting malaria. In his twenty-page report on electro zone, Reed carefully gave Lazear credit for helping him."

Private William Dean, Troop B, Seventh U.S. Cavalry also volunteered to become a test subject. These first experiments were replicated at Camp Lazear, a military post consisting of seven tents and two 14 by 20 foot frame buildings. Private John E. Kissinger and John J. Moran, a civilian clerk, were among the first to volunteer themselves as test subjects. Reed had been authorized by General Leonard Wood, military governor of Cuba, to pay one hundred dollars in gold to each test subject with an additional bonus of another hundred for subjects who contracted the disease while serving in this test. Kissinger spoke for himself and fellow volunteers when he refused the reward, saying that he participated in the study, 'solely in the interest of humanity and the cause of science.' Reed touched his cap and replied respectfully, 'Gentlemen, I salute you.'

With Lazear dead, Carroll ill and Agramonte on leave, the responsibility for the yellow fever project was now primarily Reed's concern. The results of Dean's test were reproduced again in a controlled environment. Writer captures some of the drama of this time as he describes the culmination of Dr. Reed's research. "On December 21, infected mosquitoes were released into one side of the Infected Mosquito Building, in which all items had been disinfected with steam. James Moran, who seemed determined to get yellow fever, entered the infested side of the building, while two other volunteers entered the mosquito-free side. On Christmas morning, Moran finally contracted a non-fatal case of the disease. As 1900 drew to a close, Walter Reed proudly wrote to his wife that he and his assistants had lifted 'the impenetrable veil that surrounded the causation of this most wonderful, dreadful pest of humanity . . . the prayer that has been mine for twenty years, that I might be permitted in some way or at some time to do something good to alleviate human suffering has been granted! A thousand Happy New Years."

The New Year brought Reed public recognition and private grief. Bean writes, "On September 6, 1901, William McKinley, the president of the United States, was shot by an assassin in Buffalo, New York, during the week the American Public Health Association was meeting in that city. Walter Reed was about to present his paper on 'The Prevention of Yellow Fever' when the event took place, and several of his friends and at least one of his enemies were among the consultants who hovered over the fallen president until he died on September 14."

The report that made Reed famous included the names of the other board members as co-authors. Colin Norman writes in an

article for Science magazine that Carter and Finlay were given full credit in their advisory capacity. Reed died of appendicitis in 1902. Crosby and Haubrich suggest in an article for the Journal of the American Medical Association that Reed's appendix had been weakened by previous illness, possibly cholera. These authors report that the day before Reed's death a close friend, Major Jefferson Randolph Kean, attempted to cheer Reed by saying Reed was certain to receive a promotion in the near future. Reed is said to have replied, 'I care nothing for that now.' Crosby and Haubrich indicate that during the last two years of his life Walter Reed struggled with depression brought about by a sense of guilt at having prospered at the expense of other people's suffering. He believed that the principle of informed consent did not absolve him of his share of moral responsibility for an experiment that risked human life. Reed wrote the surgeon general, "The responsibility for the life of a human weighs upon me very heavily just at present, and I am dreadfully melancholic." Walter Reed was haunted by this sense of responsibility for the rest of his life. According to Crosby and Haubrich, Lazear kept a diary while stationed in Cuba. After Lazear's death, Reed kept this diary in his personal possession in the top drawer of his office desk. This diary disappeared shortly after Walter Reed's death. He died on November 23, 1902. During his last few days, Reed obstinately postponed medical treatment that might have saved his life.
All the above according to Howard Kelly's scholarly biography.

Even today, we keep citronella oil handy for when we work outside in the garden where those buzzing insects will attack you for a sip of blood whenever they feel inclined to do so. Citronella is an effective deterrent; applying a drop or two behind the ears, arms and legs.

Schweitzer, Another great doctor

His name is in the gallery of the great ones of the world. The saga of Dr. Albert Schweitzer's personal life has deeply moved several generations not only in Europe but also in South Africa whence we came. Especially in Church circles and Sunday school at large. He was born in 1875 in Gunsbach where he was raised in both German and French culture, since his hometown was near the border of France. Now that is to say predominantly Protestant Germans and Roman faith French mingled in an unusual tolerant fashion. His father was a Reformed pastor. The family was deeply musical; both his grandfathers were well known organists. This doctor, a man of unshakable faith, truly lived up to the Hippocratic oath to the minutest detail.

German discipline and endurance, added to that his natural gifts, and I am sure encouraging parents, earned Albert a brilliant academic career. One can justifiably say that whatever he touched turned into gold. At Strasbourg in 1898 he earned a PhD with a thesis on the religious philosophy of Kant. During the same year he earned the Doctorate in Divinity. Being appointed to a position of professor was to no one's surprise.

He studied music of the organ under maestro Charles Marie Widor in Paris. Maestro Widor was one of the greatest in his time. To no one's surprise, Albert surpassed Widor in the interpretation of Johan Sebastian Bach. During all this flood of success, Schweitzer remained pre-occupied with the suffering of others. At the age of 21 Albert made his famous decision that he would live for science and art only till the age of thirty, then thereafter he would devote his life to serving his LORD and fellow man and particularly those suffering from diseases. He set his mind on studying medicine and earned his qualification as a general practitioner medical doctor.

Then, at the beginning of 1913 he received his M.D. after he had served as professor at the university of Strasbourg. He was a recipient of many awards, including the Nobel Prize. He served as a deacon in his church. In June 1912 he married Helene Bresslau, daughter of the Jewish pan-Germanist historian Harry Bresslau. In 1912, now armed with a medical degree, Schweitzer made a definite proposal to go as a medical doctor to work <u>at his own expense</u> in the Paris Missionary Society's mission at Lambaréné on the Ogooué river, in what is now the Gabon in Africa (then a French colony).

In the first nine months he and his wife had about 2,000 patients to examine, some traveling many days and hundreds of kilometers to reach him. In addition to injuries he was often treating severe sandflea and crawcraw sores (washing with mercuric chloride, framboesia (using arseno-benzol injections), tropical eating sores (cleaning and potassium permanganate, heart disease (treated with digitalin, tropical dysentery (emetine (syrup of ipecac) and arseno-benzol), tropical malaria (quinine and Arrhenal arsenic), sleeping sickness, treated at that time with atoxyl, leprosy (chaulmoogra oil), fevers, strangulated hernias (surgery), necrosis, abdominal tumors and chronic constipation and nicotine poisoning, while also attempting to deal with deliberate poisonings, fetishism and fear of cannibalism among the Mbahouin.

Mrs. Helene Schweitzer was anesthetist for surgical operations, using chloroform and Papaveretum, a synthesized morphine derivative. After briefly occupying a shed formerly used as a chicken hut, in autumn 1913 they built their first hospital of corrugated iron, with two 13-foot rooms (consulting room and operating theatre) and with a dispensary and sterilizing room in spaces below the broad eaves. The waiting room and dormitory (42 by 20 feet) were built like native huts, of unhewn logs, along a 30-yard path leading from the hospital to the landing-place. The Schweitzers had their own bungalow, and employed as their assistant Joseph, a French-speaking Galoa (Mpongwe) who first came as a patient.

When World War I broke out in summer of 1914, Schweitzer and his wife, being Germans in a French colony, were put under supervision at Lambaréné (where work continued) by the French military. In 1917, exhausted by over four years work and by tropical anemia, they went home for a short period.

He penned many books and ever made time to send his notes on his experiences to friends innumerable. I take liberty to quote from his writings, his and his wife's unselfish life experiences and battles with diseases, and in this case in particular the —glossina palpalis;— Tsetse fly that carried the Sleeping sickness‖ in a part of the world where human flesh on the menu is much sought after. In Equatorial Africa where they spent almost all of their lives, there was no McDonalds, grocery stores, paved roads, in fact no highways, but bush, bananas and savages; not to mention dangerous wild beast and snakes. There was no infrastructure of any kind. That was how it has been since creation. The Negro folks had been there since time immemorial or at least since they were driven from Canaan.

<u>From his diary and widely publicized notes:</u>

—On Good Friday in1913 the Church Bells tolled for the last time, at least for my dear wife and I when the train appeared around the corner of the woods in my native village Gunsbach in the Vosges. On this serene morning we heard once more the dear old organ of S. Sulpice's Church, and the wonderful playing of our friend Widor. This day that we finally left on our journey to the jungle seemed a glorious dream.

Among those that we got to know real well, were a lieutenant and a government official. Last mentioned had already been in Tonquin, Madagascar, Senegal, the Niger and Congo for a long time on colonial affairs. He held crushing views about Mohammedanism as it prevails among the natives, seeing in it the greatest danger there is for the future of Africa. _The Mohammedan Negro' he said, _is no longer good for anything. You may build him railways, dig them canals, and spend millions of pounds to provide irrigation for the land you hope he would cultivate. But it all makes no impression on him; he is absolutely opposed to anything European however advantageous and profitable it may be. And that is how it has been since time immemorial.'

What was very valuable to me is my acquaintance with a military doctor who already had twelve years of military experience in

Equatorial Africa, and was going to Grand Basam as director of the Bacteriological Institute there. At my request, he spared me two hours every morning, during which he gave me an account of the general system of tropical medicine, illustrated by his own experiments and experiences. He thought that it was very necessary that as many independent doctors as possible should devote themselves to the care of the native populations; only so could we hope to get the mastery of sleeping sickness.‖

What is sleeping sickness? Rest assured that it is nothing like what Rip van Winkle experienced; I after all, he at least woke up again; that is to say in this life.

The doctor writes: Sleeping sickness prevails more widely here that what I first expected. The chief focus of infection is, for now, on the Ngounje district. The Ngounje being a contributory of the Ogowe, about ninety miles from here, but there are isolated centers round Lambarene and on the lakes behind N'Gomo.

I do not intend to endeavor an autobiography of this great doctor, but merely provide some high lights on one of mankind's greatest. How on earth he still could find the time to have sent memos to many people amidst a heavy load of work baffles my mind. However, thanks to the invention of David Gestetner, a Hungarian that gave him the first real copying machine for which he earned a patent as early as 1881. Let me correct myself; saying —this great man,‖ I should say —this great couple‖. What a wife!

In my youth, I worked in the cinema theatre as operator where I saw numerous movies, amongst which were —Stanley and Dr. Livingston.‖ It ever left me wondering why those old missionaries invariably wore white clothes in the jungle. Now I know and doctor Schweitzer gives the answer in his following notes:

The doctor writes about the Tsetse Fly: What is sleeping the sickness? How is it spread? It seems to have existed since time immemorial, but it was confined to particular centers, since there was little or no traveling. From my window I can see where the N'counje enters the Ogowe River, and so far may the Galoas living around Lambarene travel. Anyone that went beyond this point father into the interior was eaten. Sleeping sickness can wipe out entire community; whenever it gets into a community it is very destructive and may carry off as much as a third of the population. In Uganda for example, it reduced the inhabitants in six years from 300,000 to 100,1000. An officer told me that he once visited a village on the upper Ogowe, which had two thousand inhabitants. On passing it again two years later, he could only count 500; the rest had meanwhile died of sleeping sickness. For reasons we cannot yet explain, the disease loses its virulence after some time.

Still close study reveals the fact that sleeping sickness can be also conveyed by mosquitoes if these insects take their blood from a healthy person immediately after they had bitten anyone with sleeping sickness, as they will then have trypanosomes in their saliva; thus the mosquito army continue by night the work which the glossina is carrying all day. Poor Africa!

In its essential nature sleeping sickness is a chronic inflammation of the meninges and the brain, one, however, which always ends in death, and this ensues because the trypanosomes pass from blood into the cerebro-spinal fluid. To fight the disease successfully, it is necessary to kill them before they have passed from the blood, since it is only that atoxyl, one weapon that we at present possess, produces effects that can to any extent be relied on; in the cerebro-spinal marrow the trypanosomes are comparatively safe from it. A doctor must therefore learn to recognize the disease in the early stage when it first produces fever. If he can do that, there is a prospect of recovery.

In the district, therefore, where sleeping sickness has to be treated, its diagnosis is a terribly complicated business because the significance of every attack of fever, of every persistent headache, of every prolonged attack of sleeping sickness, and of all rheumatic pains must be gauged with the help of the microscope. More over, the examination of the blood is, unfortunately, by no means simple, but takes a great deal of time, for it is only very seldom that these pale, thin, parasites, about eighteen thousandth [1/18,000] of a millimeter long, are to be found in a considerable number in the blood. So far, I have only examined one case in which three or four were seen together.

I must however, in justice, add that the mosquito does not harbor the trypanosomes permanently, and that its saliva is only poisonous for a short time after the blood of a sleeping sickness victim has polluted it.

—If we in our own strength confide, the battle is lostǁ, thus I quote one more paragraph from this saintly doctor's writings: Another operation is finished, and in the hardly lighted dormitory I watched for the sick man's awakening. Scarcely has he recovered consciousness when he stares about him and ejaculates again and again: —I _have no more pain! I've no more pain! …. His hand feels for mine and will not let it go. Then I begin to tell him and the others that are in the room that it is the LORD Jesus the Christ who has told the doctor and his wife to come to Ogowe, and that white people in Europe give them the money to come and cure the sick Negroes. This is when the words of Matthew xxiii verse 8 gets meaning. Would that my generous friends in Europe could come out here and live through one such hour! Sunrise brings the Tsetse Fly which is active only during daytime and compared with which the worst mosquito is a comparatively harmless creature. It is about half the size of the ordinary housefly, which it resembles in appearance; only its wings, when closed, lie parallel on the body, but overlap like the blades of a pair of scissors. For this tiny creature to get blood, it can pierce the thickest cloth. It is extremely cautious and artful, and evades cleverly all blows of the hands. The moment it feels the body on which it sits makes the slightest movement, it flies off and hides itself like on the side of the canoe. Its flight is audible. A small flywhisk is a handy weapon of defense. Its habit of caution makes it avoid settling on any light color object on which it could easily detected: hence white clothes are the best protection against it. This statement I found fully confirmed for both of us wore white only. We hardly ever had a fly making a landing on us, but the blacks were the worst sufferers.

We that take our comfortable lifestyle as an entitlement need to give it some thought as to what it took our pioneers and forefathers to pave the way for us. As much as those great missionaries had courage and faith; this old world was as wild as could come when they first ventured into this part of the world, which was as wild as the African jungle.

From the doctor's notes:

142

Another thing that worked toward our detriment was that all one's servants, even the best of them, are so unreliable that they must not be exposed to the slightest temptation. This means that they must never be left alone in the house. All the time they are at work, there my wife must be there too, and anything that might be attractive to their dishonesty must be under lock and key. Even to the cook we have to give only the right amounts of rice, potatoes etc. What is not locked up goes for a walk. Mr. Rambaud of Samkita lost in this way, part of a valuable work in several volumes, and there disappeared one day from my bookshelf the piano addition of Wagner's —Meister Singer‖ and the copy of Bach's Passion Music [St. Matthew,] into which I had written the accompaniment, which I had worked out very carefully. This feeling of never being safe from their stupidest piece of theft, brings one sometimes almost to despair, and to have to keep everything locked up and turn oneself into a walking bunch of keys, adds a terrible burden on life.

The African sun is shining through the coffee bushes into the dark shed, but we, black and white, sit side by side and feel that we know by experience the meaning of the words of St. Matthew 23 verse 8.

Dr. Albert Schweitzer 1:14: 1875-- 9:4:1965

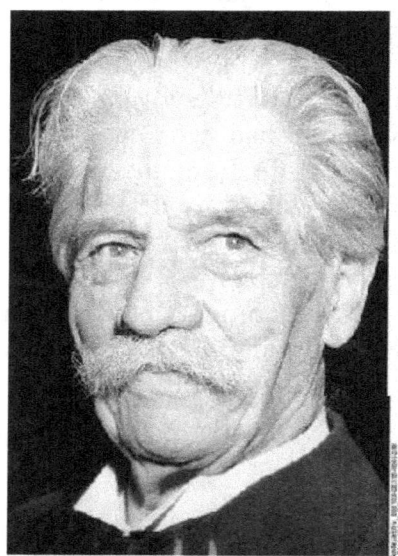

Dr. Albert Schweitzer, the humanitarian, theologian, missionary, organist, and medical doctor and philosopher Nobel Prize winner and more. After retiring as a practicing doctor, Albert Schweitzer continued to oversee the hospital until his death at the age of 90.

People listen to people.

It always fascinates me to watch people react to the news broadcast, and how easily they become influenced by what they hear. But what really is amazing me is how people are persuaded by a smooth talker and believe what they hear as gospel. The belief system of an entire generation can be turned around by a handful of intelligent men deceived by their own preconceptions that had totally blinded them from the truth. All in all, and very unfortunate, so many of us are not really interested in considering fiction and facts critically; not ascertaining the possibilities and impossibilities. Only recently we witnessed the uprising in Libya and Egypt, that evidently got started by a couple of frustrated young Moslems, influenced by members of the Inter-Arab states Moslem Brotherhood, went running down the street chanting well-prepared caliphate indoctrinated slogans, and before long it grew into a large crowd and eventually spilled over to other Arab states. With such kind of demonstrators one can ask them individually what they are doing there; invariably the answer would be —Oh I don't know, I just joined the parade.‖

This sort of thing I've seen in many parts of the world; and it is not new; consider the time of the crucifixion of Messiah; there it was a priest or more that actually started the chant, so effective, and was the result that the chief civil magistrate was persuaded to convict an innocent Man; for which Pilate was eventually court martialled on the charge that he illegally crucified an innocent Man.

A very successful businessman once made a preposterous statement, saying that General Mozes thought out the Ten Commandments for aiding him in controlling a couple million of unruly Israelites. Now this statement was made to me in private conversation; so what would have happened should I have accepted that nonsense as truth? Even worse, if I had built a thesis on that; my reaction to this very well educated lawyer was simply, —You are playing with fire my friend, and you may very well get burnt.‖

What I am trying to convey to my readers is simply this: If any man from that pulpit or anywhere else, tells you that the eating of the forbidden food, according to the New Testament is legal, then consider the consequences and the facts that are clearly spelled out in the Maker's Handbook wherein the Almighty Yahweh never once contradicts Himself.

Once again the Old Maker's Handbook has it so right where it says in Proverbs 12:15. The way of a fool is right in his own eyes: but he that hearkeneth unto counsel is wise.

Now, my prayer for you is a healthy and happy life.

Cheerio.

When I was one-and-twenty
I heard a wise man say
—Give crowns and pounds and
Guineas
But not your heart away:
Give pearls away and rubies
But keep your fancy free."
But I was one-and-twenty,
No use to talk to me.
From A.E. Houseman.

Ps. I was just wondering about them locusts, frogs, and flies and flees; may be the residue of Pharaoh's disobedience?